KU-246-123

Monoclonal antibody technology

LABORATORY TECHNIQUES IN BIOCHEMISTRY AND MOLECULAR BIOLOGY

Volume 13

Edited by

R.H. BURDON - *Department of Biochemistry, University of Glasgow*

P.H. van KNIPPENBERG - *Department of Biochemistry, University of Leiden*

Advisory board

P. BORST - *University of Amsterdam*
D.C. BURKE - *University of Warwick*
P.B. GARLAND - *University of Dundee*
M. KATES - *University of Ottawa*
W. SZYBALSKI - *University of Wisconsin*
H.G. WITTMAN - *Max-Planck Institut für Molekuläre Genetik, Berlin*

ELSEVIER
AMSTERDAM · NEW YORK · OXFORD

MONOCLONAL ANTIBODY TECHNOLOGY

THE PRODUCTION AND CHARACTERIZATION OF RODENT AND HUMAN HYBRIDOMAS

Ailsa M. Campbell

Department of Biochemistry,
University of Glasgow, Glasgow G12 8QQ (Great Britain)

1984

ELSEVIER
AMSTERDAM · NEW YORK · OXFORD

1984, Elsevier Science Publishers B.V.

All rights reserved. No part of this publication may be reproduced, stored in a retrieval system, or transmitted, in any form or by any means, mechanical, photocopying, recording or otherwise, without the prior permission of the copyright owner. However, this book has been registered with the Copyright Clearance Center, Inc. Consent is given for copying pages for personal of internal use of specific clients. This consent is given on the condition that the copier pay through the Center the per page fee stated below for copying beyond that permitted by the U.S. Copyright Law.

The appropriate fee should be forwarded with a copy of front and back of the title page of the book to the Copyright Clearance Center, Salem, MA 0197). This consent does not extend to other kinds of copying, such as for general distribution, resale, advertising and promotional purposes, or for creating new works. Special written permission must be obtained from the publisher for such copying.

The per page fee code for this book is 0-444-80575-3 (pocket edition): 84/$0.80; 0-444-80592-3 (library edition): 84/$0.80. series: 0-7204-4200-1: 84/$0.80.

ISBN 0-444-80575-3 (pocket edition)
    0-444-80592-3 (library edition)
    series: 0-7204-4200-1

Published by:
ELSEVIER SCIENCE PUBLISHERS B.V.
PO BOX 211
1000 AE AMSTERDAM
THE NETHERLANDS

Sole distributors for the USA and Canada:
ELSEVIER SCIENCE PUBLISHING COMPANY, INC.
52 VANDERBILT AVENUE
NEW YORK, NY 10017
USA

Library of Congress Cataloging in Publication Data

Campbell, Ailsa M.
    Monoclonal antibody technology.

    Includes index.
    1. Antibodies, Monoclonal. 2. Hybridomas.
3. Biotechnology. I. Title. [DNLM: 1. Antibodies,
Monoclonal. 2. Hybidomas. 3. Immunologic Technics.
W1 LA232K v.13 / QW 575 C187m]
QR186.85.C36 1984   615'.37   84-10322
ISBN 0-444-80592-3
ISBN 0-444-80575-3 (pbk.)

This book is the pocket edition of Volume 13, of the series 'Laboratory Techniques in Biochemistry and Molecular Biology'

Printed in The Netherlands

Preface

This book is essentially a laboratory manual based on the protocols and general advice currently available in our own department. It was written, for the two groups of people who have consulted us extensively over the past few years. The first were competent biochemists who were interested in the potential of monoclonal antibodies as reagents either to study basic biochemistry or to develop better clinical assay systems. The second were clinicians with an interest in the potential of monoclonal antibodies for the detection and potential therapy of various clinical conditions who had sufficient technical assistance to feel that they might embark on monoclonal antibody production themselves using material from their own patients.

The main questions raised by discussions with these two groups were related to the possibility of obtaining the monoclonal antibody (or panel of monoclonal antibodies) required in a period of $1-2$ years or indeed at all. Many of the general multi-author review articles written by those who had been successful give the impression that monoclonal antibodies may be produced against any epitope of any molecule, however impure and the practical problems that such an approach might encounter had to be analysed. An example might be, how sensible is it to try and raise a panel of human monoclonal antibodies to a tumour of limited allogeneic cross reaction, of which samples are available at a level of 10^7 tumour cells every six months. Another might be the practicability of raising rodent monoclonal antibodies to a molecule which is only available in a highly impure state. A third might be the likelihood of making rodent monoclonal antibodies of a chosen specificity and affinity to a small peptide hormone. Many of the projects suggested seemed unlikely to succeed for technical reasons while some had considerable potential. The book attempts to guide the reader through what may be possible and what is less likely to succeed in the limited time period available to most laboratories.

Those projects which had the most potential and were initiated then required that detailed protocols be available to the personnel involved. In particular, advice on tissue culture techniques, immunisation and animal handling, failures in growth and/or antibody secretion and the potential idiosyncrasies of monoclonal antibodies in assay and purification was sought. The book incorporates the accumulated experience of our own and other laboratories in this respect.

Glasgow, June 1984   AILSA M. CAMPBELL

Acknowledgements

Many people have contributed to this book. In particular I should like to thank Marion Mc Cormack, Jacki Bennett and Souravi Ghosh who have been invaluable colleagues in the laboratory and Ian Ramsden and his staff in the Glasgow University Medical Illustration Unit who have been responsible for the illustrations. Janet Jones not only wrote Appendix I but taught us most of the techniques described in it.

I am also indebted to Caroline Addey, Flora Campbell, Magnus Campbell, John Coggins, Dorothy Crawford, Bertil Damato, Morag Davidson, Jim Dunn, Christopher Edwards, Malcolm Ferguson Smith, Frank Fleming, Robin Fraser, Angus Munro, Rosalind Quinn, Celia Ross, Asaad Shallal, Martin Smellie, Elizabeth Smith, Alan Williamson and Veronica van Heyningen for information, support or advice. In addition, I thank the Glasgow University Biochemistry secretariat for help in word processing.

Abbreviations

EB	Epstein Barr
ELISA	Enzyme linked immunosorbent assay
G banding	Staining of chromosomes with Giemsa stain
HAT	Hypoxanthine, aminopterin and thymidine
HT	Hypoxanthine and thymidine
IRMA	Immunoradiometric assay
PAGE	Polyacrylamide gel electrophoresis
PEG	Polyethylene glycol
SDS	Sodium dodecyl sulphate

Contents

General properties and applications of monoclonal antibodies

1.1. Introduction

The technique of cell hybridisation or fusion has been applied to a large number of problems in the biomedical sciences. It has proved to be a major tool in determining which human chromosome codes for a specific gene function by means of the analysis of the isoenzyme patterns produced by a panel of clones from human–rodent fusions (Ruddle and Kucherlapali, 1974). In addition, it has been used to characterise the dominant or recessive nature of malignancy by means of fusion of normal cells with malignant cells (Harris, 1970; Croce and Kaprowski, 1974). In the early days the fusion agent, or fusogen, was an inactivated virus, most commonly sendai virus (Harris and Watkins, 1965). However, in recent years the use of chemical fusogens such as polyethylene glycol (PEG) has become more common (Pontecorvo, 1976). The production of monoclonal antibodies remains only one of the many applications of the technique and it is likely that cell hybridisation will be used extensively in the long term for the immortalisation of many other differentiated cell functions and that the extensive practical experience developed in the optimisation of hybridoma production may lead to the expansion of the application of cell fusion techniques in other areas (Ringertz and Savage, 1976).

The theory of monoclonal antibody production is based on the clonal selection hypothesis of Macfarlane Burnet (Burnet, 1959). Each mammalian B lymphocyte has the potential to make a mono-specific antibody. The constant region of the antibody chain may alter during the differentiation of the lymphocyte clone but the variable region retains this singular specificity. Recent research in immunogenetics has shown that the origin of this specificity is complex and involves not only the extensive rearrangement of the DNA sequences in the chromosomes which code for the antibody chains but also some degree of somatic mutation during clonal development (reviewed by Tonegawa, 1983). The broader immunological background can be found in several recent textbooks (McConnell, Munro and Waldman, 1981; Roitt, 1980; Weissman, Hood and Wood, 1978). Weir (1978) is the most comprehensive methodology text.

The first report of hybridoma production was in fact in 1970 (Sinkovics et al., 1970) with virus specific lymphocytes together with tumour cells and subsequent reports of both interspecies (Schwaber and Cohen, 1973) and human (Bloom and Nakamura, 1974) hybridomas appeared in the literature before the full potential of the technology was expanded by Kohler and Milstein in 1975. Since then there has been exponential growth in the literature relating to monoclonal antibody production and utilisation.

The experimental problem encountered in monospecific antibody production relates to the fact that plasma cells which secrete antibody are terminally differentiated lymphocytes with a finite lifespan. They cannot normally be grown in culture. However, tumours of such cells can be found in most animals and, in particular, can be readily induced in mice with the aid of mineral oils. The tumour cells secrete an antibody of single, unknown and almost certainly unwanted specificity but can grow indefinitely in culture. Consequently, if such tumour cells can be fused with a lymphocyte which makes antibody of the required specificity, the progeny may have the eternal growth capacity of one parent together with the specific antibody production capacity of the other (Kohler and Milstein, 1975, 1976). Essentially a refinement of the technique involves the selection of a mutant strain of the tumour parent line which does not itself secrete antibody so that the production capacity of the progeny is directed to the specific antibody. A further sophistication, which is more essential, is to select a parent line which is in some way vulnerable to the cell culture conditions so that it can not survive unless it has participated in a

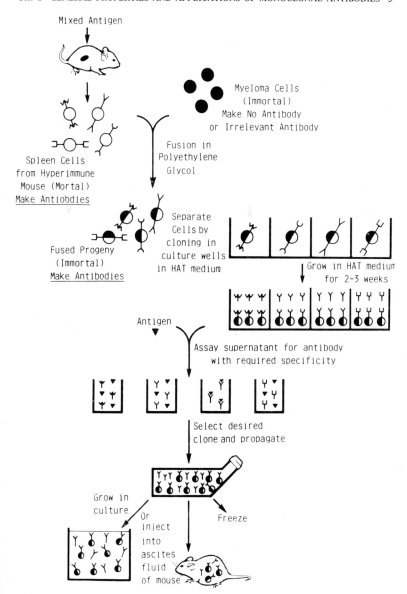

Fig. 1.1. The general procedures of monoclonal antibody production in mice.

fusion. The commonest way of achieving this is to use a parent tumour line which lacks either the enzyme thymidine kinase (TK) or hypoxanthine phosphoribosyl transferase (HPRT). These are enzymes of the salvage pathway of nucleic acid metabolism and are essential to cells growing in the presence of aminopterin which blocks the main pathways of nucleotide synthesis. After the fusion the cells are therefore usually grown on medium containing Hypoxanthine, Aminopterin and Thymidine (HAT) (Littlefield, 1964; Chapter 3) in which any parent tumour cells which have not participated in a fusion will die. Fig. 1.1 shows schematically the outline of the fusion procedure. The hybrid cells are grown in culture plates and assayed for the production of the required antibody after a suitable period of time, usually 10–14 days. Suitable clones are then selected for expansion and subcloning so that eventually the required antibody may be produced in large amounts. It is the purpose of this volume to enable the reader to undertake these procedures in his own laboratory and produce an antibody of the required immunoglobulin class, specificity and affinity. At present, the choice of animal is limited to mouse, rat or man. Several recent reviews and books specifically directed towards monoclonal antibody production have been published (Galfre and Milstein, 1981; Goding, 1980; Fazekas De St Groth and Scheiddeger, 1980; Kennet et al., 1980; Eisenbarth, 1981; Hammerling et al., 1981; McMichael and Fabre, 1982). The procedures are undergoing constant modification and the Addendum at the end of the book is intended to detail the more significant of those which occur between the time of going to press and publication.

1.2. Comparison of monoclonal antibodies and conventional antiserum

Monoclonal antibody production consumes very much more time and money than the production of conventional antiserum. It is sensible therefore to consider what advantages may be realistically gained by the use of this technique and whether conventional antiserum may not suffice for the project which is envisaged. Table 1.1 gives a comparison between the two, indicating the main advantages which may be expected from monoclonal as opposed to polyclonal antibodies of conventional antiserum. These are analysed in more detail in the sections which follow.

1.2.1. Specificity: advantages

The antigenic determinant is the particular site on the antigen (which may be a very large molecule) responsible for binding the antibody.

TABLE 1.1

Comparison between conventional serum and monoclonal antibodies

	Conventional antiserum	Monoclonal antibody
Determinant	Several	Single
Specificity	Variable with animal and bleed	Standard
	Partial cross-reactions with common determinants	Unexpected cross reactions may occur
	Seldom too specific	May be too specific for requirements
Affinity	Variable with bleed	May be selected during cloning
Yield of useful antibody	Up to 1 mg/ml	Up to 100 μg/ml in tissue culture Up to 20 mg/ml in ascitic fluid
Contaminating immunoglobulin	Up to 100%	None in culture 10% in ascitic fluid
Purity of antigen	Either pure antigen or serum absorption	Some degree of antigen purification desirable but not essential
Approximate minimum cost	Usually below £100	Capital cost £10000 Running costs £10000 p.a.

Typically, this will be a small group of amino acid or carbohydrate residues. Conventional antiserum (polyclonal) will not only have antibodies to several determinants (Fig. 1.2) but also a family of antibodies of different structure and avidity which compete for each individual determinant. Consequently extensive cross reaction may occur between antibodies and two proteins which have similar determinants. This may be avoided completely by the use of monoclonal antibodies which have been selected for their ability to bind to a determinant unique to the required antigen (Fig. 1.3). The most

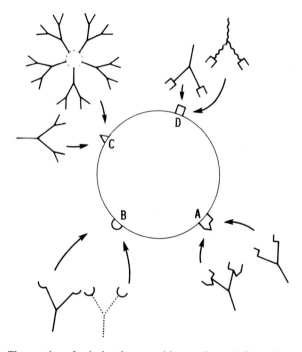

Fig. 1.2. The reaction of polyclonal serum with an antigen. At determinant A are two antibodies of the same class but different specificities and affinities. At determinant B are two antibodies of different class, specificity and affinity. At determinant C are two antibodies of different class, one being an IgM but the same affinity and specificity. At determinant D are two antibodies of different class but the same specificity and affinity.

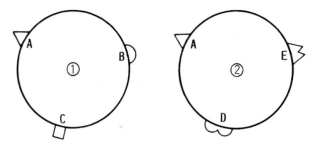

Fig. 1.3. Potential cross-reactions with two largely dissimilar antigens. Antiserum raised to antigen 1 will only show partial cross-reaction when tested with antigen 2 as determinant A is shared but the other two determinants are not. Monoclonal antibodies to determinant A will cross-react 100% with antigen 2. Monoclonal antibodies to determinants B and C will not cross-react at all with antigen 2.

refined application of the specificity is in detecting subtle antigenic differences between two strains of a bacterium or virus and utilising these differences for diagnostic or preparative purposes. Similarly, a pair of polypeptide hormones which have one chain in common and the other unique may readily be differentiated for use in radioimmunoassay, or two steroid hormones which differ by a single chemical grouping may be assayed separately. At its simplest, the high specificity of a monoclonal antibody reduces non-specific background cross-reactivity so that techniques such as immunohistochemical localisation may be very much improved.

The high degree of specificity that may be obtained with a monoclonal antibody has opened up the possibility of tumour immunotherapy, either with antibody by itself, or antibody coupled to drugs or toxins, and successful treatments of leukaemias with murine monoclonal antibodies have already been reported (Section 1.3.2). While such applications emphasise the immense potential of the specificity of monoclonal antibodies, they also emphasise the importance of understanding the possible cross reactions that may unexpectedly occur with such a tool.

1.2.2. Specificity: disadvantages

There are two main areas in which the specificity of a monoclonal antibody may be less precise than expected and where indeed cross-reactivity may be greater than that experienced with normal serum (Fig. 1.3). Firstly, the determinant may be present on other molecules which have not been tested in the screening procedure. An obvious example is with two proteins which have the same prosthetic group. If the monoclonal antibody is directed to this group and it is equally accessible in both proteins, it is possible to have 100% cross-reactivity. With conventional serum, there would be antibodies directed at determinants not common to both proteins and cross-reactivity could be very slight. The selection and testing of the monoclonal antibody should in principle be able to eliminate this difficulty but may be a complex process. While it is possible to test the antibody against antigens which are known or suspected to share common determinants, elimination of those antibodies which may display cross-reactivity to a particular cell type is a lengthy procedure. Many cell surface antigens are carbohydrates in nature and the same antigenic sites may be present on two cell types which are structurally dissimilar and functionally distant in the body (Gerson et al., 1982). While such cross-reactivity may not represent a major problem in diagnostic and preparative use, it clearly presents a major potential hazard in therapeutic use, and extensive preliminary experiments are essential. It must be emphasised that the extent to which cross-reacting determinants on molecules which have no other structural similarity exist is only now coming to light since before the discovery of monoclonal antibodies there was no methodology sensitive enough to measure it (see Lane and Koprowski, 1982 for a review).

It is also possible for an antibody selected as totally specific in one assay to cross-react extensively in another assay, especially where fixatives have been used in a primary immunocytochemical assay (Milstein et al., 1983).

A second type of cross-reactivity which may occur with monoclonal antibodies can be found where the same antibody reacts with two

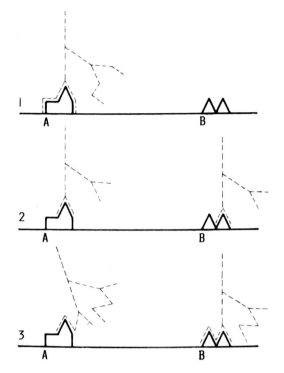

Fig. 1.4. Potential cross-reaction of single antibodies with two dissimilar determinants. In 1, the antibody is totally specific for determinant A. In 2, it has equal affinity and specificity for both A and B. In 3, it has greater specificity (and probably affinity, see text) for B but also cross-reacts with A.

totally different determinants (Fig. 1.4). The best known example of this phenomenon is evidenced by myeloma protein 460 which binds dinitrophenol lysine and methyl naphthoquinone at distinct but overlapping points. The conventional assumption that all antibodies are monospecific may therefore not be correct (Richards et al., 1975).

Cross-reactivities of the two types should not affect the majority of uses of monoclonal antibodies. However, they do emphasise the importance of the selection procedures being oriented as closely as possible towards the final application of the monoclonal antibody.

Whereas cross-reactivity may present occasional problems, at the other extreme, a monoclonal antibody may be produced which is too specific for its final application (Fig. 1.5). A typical example may be in general viral or bacterial diagnosis where the antibody reacts with a single determinant not present on all strains of the pathogen. Similarly, a monoclonal antibody cannot be used in a routine clinical radioimmunoassay of a protein which exhibits polymorphism throughout the population, unless it is certain that the antibody is directed towards an invariant determinant. Their standard nature and low background make monoclonal antibodies very attractive reagents for this type of routine immunodiagnostic use and paradoxically, it is therefore likely that the best way of obtaining a suitable reagent will be to mix two or more monoclonal antibodies directed against different epitopes on the antigen. In this way the chances of not detecting the antigen are minimised while the standard nature and low background are preserved. Further hazards of monoclonal antibody specificity relate to their very precise assay requirements. These are discussed in detail in Chapter 2. None preclude the use of the antibody, but rather influence the possibility of detecting them on the initial screening procedure.

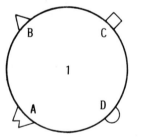 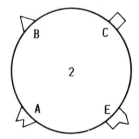

Fig. 1.5. Potential cross-reaction with two largely similar antigens. Conventional serum raised to antigen 1 will cross-react very extensively with antigen 2 as it has determinants A, B and C in common. Monoclonal antibodies directed to derminants A, B or C will cross-react 100%. However monoclonal antibodies directed to determinant D will not recognise antigen 2.

1.2.3. Affinity: advantages

Since each antigenic determinant may elicit the production of a series of antigens of variable affinity, it is possible by monoclonal antibody technology to select out an antibody of the required association constant, rejecting those of higher or lower avidity. This has obvious value in techniques such as radioimmunoassay where a high avidity antibody is generally required for maximum sensitivity and in most cases a high affinity monoclonal antibody is required and selected. However, preparative procedures often employ an antibody of lower affinity deliberately. For example, the antigen may be a protein vulnerable to denaturation by the extreme conditions required to elute it from a preparative affinity column and purification would be better handled with a low affinity monoclonal antibody where more gentle elution procedures could be applied.

The association constant between a monospecific antibody and its determinant is quantitated by the rate constants for association and for dissociation. These two parameters may vary independently of each other according to the experimental conditions. It is therefore possible in principle not only to select a monoclonal antibody of a chosen avidity but also to select one with a desired association or dissociation rate. For example, an association constant of 10^{10} l/mole may reflect an association rate of 10^5 l/mole/sec and dissociation rate of 10^{-5}/sec or an association rate of 10^3 l/mole/sec and dissociation rate of 10^{-7}/sec. The former might be more suitable for preparative procedures than the latter.

1.2.4. Affinity: disadvantages

It has often been suggested that monoclonal antibodies will never be able to replace conventional antisera as the essential high affinity of an antiserum lies in the cooperative effects between multiple types of antibody. There is some basis for this view. For example, two types of monoclonal antibody directed towards different determinants on the same molecule may be shown to enhance mutually the affinity of each other (Ehrlich et al., 1982). The mechanism of such enhancement is not clear but it is unlikely to involve allosteric changes in antigen structure. It is possible that circular complexes involving two antibody molecules of different specificity and two antigen molecules have greater stability (Fig. 1.6a). Alternatively there may be more subtle interactions between the Fc regions of the antibodies. It should however be made clear that not all pairs of monoclonal antibodies directed at different epitopes on the same antigen have synergistic effects (Fig. 6b). Furthermore many monoclonal antibodies of high avidity can have been produced so such effects either cannot be general or cannot be significant.

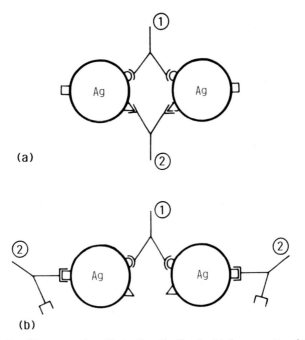

Fig. 1.6. Possible cooperative effects of antibodies. In (a) the geometry of the antigen–antibody complex is such that the two antibodies can act cooperatively stabilising the binding of each other. As a result the two antibodies together have higher affinity than would be expected from a mixture. In (b) the position of the determinants is such that cooperative binding does not occur.

In the initial selection and screening of antibodies it is extremely difficult to select for an antibody of chosen avidity. Very small amounts of antibody are available at the early stages so that the determination of the association constant is an unrealistic aim. A strongly positive result may indicate an antibody of high affinity or simply the presence of a clone secreting large amounts of antibody. A second procedure involving quantitative estimation of the amount of immunoglobulin secreted can be employed in such situations (Chapter 2; Section 10.4.7). Clones which give a strong reaction with the antigen but have little immunoglobulin are then selected for subcloning.

1.2.5. Affinity and specificity: interrelationships

It will be apparent from the preceding sections that affinity and specificity are closely linked in the selection precedures for monoclonal antibodies. It is possible to isolate a monoclonal antibody which is highly specific in the assay system used for the screening procedure only to find that it cross-reacts extensively when it is used in a more sensitive assay system. Conversely an apparently non specific antibody may be made specific under more stringent experimental conditions where only epitopes specific to the antigen are recognised (Mossman et al., 1980). The importance of the selection procedure is again emphasised and if this does not bear a close relationship to the ultimate use of the final monoclonal antibody produced, undesirable cross-reaction may occur.

1.2.6. Standardisation

As a standard reagent, a monoclonal antibody is undoubtedly superior to polyclonal serum. The latter is variant with animal and bleed so that much experimental effort must go into the standardisation of each serum sample. The animals themselves are mortal and a regular supply of purified material for immunisation is essential. Providing that there were no administrative or commercial complications, a single monoclonal antibody could be used as a diagnostic reagent throughout a wide geographical area. The only possible difficulty could lie in antigenic variation within the population as is discussed in Section 1.2.3 and this should readily be overcome by the use of a chosen mixture of monospecific antibodies.

1.2.7. Yield and purity

Monoclonal antibodies produced in tissue culture tend to give yields in the order of µg/ml. In the ascitic fluid of mice yields are greatly magnified and are in the order of mg/ml. Human hybridomas may be propagated by either method since it is possible, though difficult, to produce them in milligram quantities in nude (athymic) mice. The majority of monoclonal antibodies will grow in ascitic fluid. In principle tissue culture should yield antibody free of contaminating immunoglobulins, although the foetal calf serum employed may have up to 1.5 mg/ml bovine immunoglobulin (Chapter 9). Other contaminating proteins from the foetal calf serum will of course also be present but these may readily be removed by affinity chromatography. Ascitic fluid may have a small amount of contamination from mouse serum, the irrelevant immunoglobulin content being more difficult to remove as it it is from the same species. While the yield of conventional serum in terms of antibody may be of the same order of magnitude the contamination with irrelevant immunoglobulin is very much greater and the monoclonal system is therefore again superior.

1.2.8. Purification requirements

In the production of conventional antiserum there are two conventional methods of preparing antibodies specific to a single antigen. The most common is to purify the antigen before immunisation of the animal. However, it is also possible to absorb the serum produced so that antibodies which cross-react with undesired components of the original mixture may be removed. Antigen purification may be a very time consuming task and absorption procedures are frequently unsatisfactory yielding low and highly variable titres. In theory, monoclonal antibody production does not require a pure antigen since the appropriate antibody is selected from the cloned culture. Thus it is possible to produce an antibody to a minor component of a complex mixture which was itself impossible or very hard to purify by conventional biochemical techniques. This has indeed been achieved with spectacular success in the case of alpha interferon (Secher and Burke, 1980). In this respect monoclonal antibodies may be said to be greatly superior to conventional antisera. However two points should be made. The first is that in order to select a clone secreting the specific antibody a certain amount of pure antigen is required at some stage unless a bioassay can be established. Once the monoclonal antibody has been isolated, pure antigen may be produced by affinity chromatography so that frequently research laboratories find themselves in this 'chicken and egg' situation. Secondly, in practice most fusion products reflect the immunodominance of the serum antibodies. If the immunising mixture contains a large number of strong antigens then these will tend to mask the minor antigenic components and the number of clones which produce antibody reacting with the minor antigens is greatly reduced. Some sort of preliminary purification of the antigen is therefore highly desirable and one method of accomplishing this is by sequential fusions where the major antigens are selected out and removed from the immunising mixture by their own monoclonal antibodies. Consequently while it may be true in general to say that no purification procedures are required, this may not be true in practice with any specific antigenic mixture (see Chapter 4).

1.2.9. Selection of immunoglobulin isotype

For certain uses of antibodies it is desirable to select for or against a certain type of immunoglobulin. For example antibodies which specifically do or not react with Fc receptors may be desirable in the final application, or the multivalence of IgM molecules may be considered an advantage in, say, a complement fixation assay. Suitable antibodies can be readily detected in the panel of hybridomas produced by the appropriate assay typing at an early stage in the procedure (Chapter 3), by the use of selected tissues for fusion, or by selective immunisation (Chapter 4). It is, however, becoming apparent that the general properties which were attributed to such antibodies in studies with conventional sera do not always extrapolate to monoclonal ones. For example not all IgM monoclonal antibodies will fix complement and many IgG ones do not. Furthermore, it is becoming apparent that while the multivalence of IgM antibodies may be considered to increase assay sensitivity, in general such antibodies appear to be of lower affinity (Rodwell et al., 1983).

1.2.10. Cost

The cost of production of conventional antiserum is undoubtedly very much lower than that of producing a monoclonal antibody. While typical production costs are shown in Table 1.1 these are inevitably subject to many variable factors. A mouse or rat monoclonal antibody to a dominant antigen could be produced by an experienced operator in a well equipped laboratory in a few months. The same operator could be responsible for a variety of antigens provided that the experiments were arranged to minimise overlap. This would also be time saved by the reduced requirements for purifying the primary antigen or absorbing the serum. On the more pessimistic side, a laboratory which had no previous experience and was obliged to purchase the appropriate tissue culture apparatus and develop their own expertise would take considerably longer at much greater expense. If, in addition, they were obliged to undertake sequential monoclonal antibody production in order to isolate a minor component of a highly antigenic mixture, the time involved and the running costs would be very extensive.

If a single hybridoma line is all that is required then collaborative work with a laboratory with the appropriate facilities and experience would generally be the better course of action. More detailed costing information is given in Chapter 5.

1.3. Applications of monoclonal antibodies

The applications of monoclonal antibody technology are generally outwith the scope of this volume and are reviewed in several others (McMichael and Fabre, 1982; Albertini and Ekins, 1981; Hammerling, Hammerling and Kearney, 1981; Kennett, McKearn and Bechtol, 1980; Edwards, 1981; Yelton and Scharff, 1981). The *Index Medicus* lists several hundred papers each month under the heading of monoclonal antibodies. It is, however, possible to outline some of the major applications of monoclonal antibody technology at the present time so that the range and scope of the technique may be summarised.

1.3.1. Diagnostic uses

Antibodies produced in the mouse or the rat are most commonly used for diagnostic purposes as they are more readily produced. Not only is the fusion frequency an order of magnitude higher but the animal can be hyperimmunised with the chosen antigen. The major advantage of monoclonal antibodies over conventional sera in this application is probably their ready availability for an indefinite period at a standard titre, making direct comparisons between different laboratories comparatively simple. However, their high specificity has added greatly to the accuracy and speed of the diagnosis. Thus antibodies to common serum analytes such as protein hormones or alphafetoprotein are already commercially marketed and are slowly replacing conventional sera.

A very large number of monoclonal antibodies have been produced to a wide range of viruses such as influenza (Gerhard et al., 1981), hepatitis (Shih et al., 1980; Wands et al., 1981), polio (Ferguson et al., 1981; 1982), Epstein Barr virus (Hoffman et al., 1980) and rabies (Wiktor and Koprowski, 1978). Their high specificity has led to accurate identification between similar strains of virus such as Herpes simplex Types I and II (Pereira et al., 1980; Zweig et al., 1979). They may also be used for early diagnosis of the IgM production in affected patients. On a more basic level of research, it has been possible to make detailed charts of the antigenic drift which occurs in viruses such as influenza. Work in this area has clearly emphasised some of the problems of overspecificity referred to above in that variants which do not react with a single monoclonal antibody are readily isolated and such an antibody would clearly be unsuitable for wide ranging diagnostic purposes. Already, panels of monoclonal antibodies which are selected so that all known variants of a viral infection may be detected have been produced (Richman et al., 1981).

Antibodies designed to perform a similar function with bacterial diseases are plentiful though less common. Their applications are broadly similar and the high specificity should prove particularly helpful in the analysis of bacterial spores which tend to show extensive cross-reactivity in conventional immunological analysis. In addition, monoclonal antibodies to bacterial toxins have been generated (Remmers et al., 1982; Kozbor et al., 1982).

The considerable potential of monoclonal antibodies in the study of parasitic diseases has already been widely exploited in the most common ones such as malaria (Yoshida et al., 1980; Rener et al., 1980), schistosomiasis (Taylor and Butterworth, 1982; Smith et al., 1982) and leishmania (McMahon-Pratt and David, 1981). The advantages here are not only the obvious diagnostic ones but also that the study of the disease itself may be undertaken in greater depth since many different surface antigens may be expressed at varying stages of the life cycle of the parasite (see Rowe, 1980 for a review).

Immunological tissue typing has been a diagnostic area in which large amounts of reliable reagents at high titre have long since been required. Until recently such identification has depended on sera from multiple blood transfusion recipients, multiparous women or volunteers, and extensive adsorption has been required so that low and variable titres are produced. Monoclonal antibodies which may be used in tissue typing are now being produced by several laboratories (Brodsky et al., 1979; Trucco et al., 1979; Howard et al., 1979).

Tumour diagnosis is undoubtedly the field in which there has been most interest in monoclonal antibodies at the present time. There has been much interest in the possible general use of antibodies which react solely with tumour associated antigens and can consequently be used as wide ranging diagnostic tools (Ashall et al., 1982; McGee et al., 1982). However, antibodies to tissue or cell type specific antigens are more readily generated and these have great potential in the detection of tumours and their metastases. Monoclonal antibodies have been generated against a wide variety of lymphocyte cell surface antigens (reviewed in Janossy, 1982; Janossy et al., 1982), epithelial cells (Taylor-Papadimitrou et al., 1981; Epenetos et al., 1982b). In addition, monoclonal antibodies of high affinity will probably prove superior in the detection of tumour markers in the serum of affected patients. The range of immunochemical techniques involved in this major area of application is wide including immunocytochemistry (McGee et al., 1982), scintigraphy (Epenetos et al., 1982), radioimmunoassay and various solid phase techniques among the most common. It is evident that the monoclonal antibodies are not only used for detection of the primary tumour but also for the monitoring of the progress of the disease and of the effects of therapy. It is, however, worth noting that unexpected cross-reactivities may confuse the results. Thus monoclonal antibodies which showed intitial apparent total specificity for certain differentiation stages of T lymphocytes were subsequently shown to cross react extensively with Purkinje neurones (Gerson et al., 1982).

The techniques largely developed for the detection of primary and secondary tumour growth may of course be used in the study of other diseased states where abnormal tissue or serum components are a characteristic feature and there has been considerable interest in the fields of cardiology (Haber et al., 1982), autoimmune disease, metabolic malfunction and general laboratory immunoassay procedures.

There are diagnostic applications in which human monoclonal antibodies are the preferred tool and may become more widespread in their use as their production becomes easier. The advantage in some of these applications is self evident such as in scintigraphy where there is a danger of antispecies antibodies being produced in the patient if frequent scans are required. However, human antibodies may also be employed in the study of the nature of the immune response to disease being mounted by the patient. In tumour diagnosis this can give an indication of the extent to which the patient has been able too mount a response to the disease at different stages of progression and there is much information to be obtained by amplifying this response in vitro. There is also considerable interest in the potential amplification and analysis of the immune response in autoimmune disease (Schoenfeld et al., 1982, 1983). Small serum samples do not readily yield a high enough titre for the full spectrum of antibodies produced by the patient to be identified but monoclonal antibody production can again amplify the response in vitro. The range of epitopes within a group of patients may also be studied. In this context it is interesting to note the increasing use of Epstein Barr virus to transform the peripheral blood lymphocytes. EB virus has the considerable advantage of transforming most of the B lymphocytes in a sample thus increasing the probability of detecting those lymphocytes producing autoantibodies which are as yet uncharacterised (Kozbor and Roder, 1981; Steinitz et al., 1980).

1.3.2. Therapeutic uses

The majority of therapeutic applications of monoclonal antibodies to date have involved those raised in a mouse (Ritz et al., 1981; Miller et al., 1981, 1982; Beverley, 1982). This is largely because of the considerable problems that have been encountered in the production of human monoclonal antibodies and it is likely that as these difficulties are resolved human antibodies will have much wider use. Murine antibodies have the obvious disadvantage of being foreign to the human system and likely therefore to lose their efficacy on continual application as a host response is mounted. In addition, the host response in itself may be harmful to the patient leading to serum sickness. While there are comparatively few situations in which the treatment with the monoclonal antibodies may be undertaken externally, the treatment of bone marrow allogeneic or autologous transplants is one such area in which murine monoclonal antibodies have been shown to be of value in either reducing graft versus host disease or in removing leukemic cells from autografts (Janossy, 1982; Janossy et al., 1982; Ritz et al., 1982; Kemshead et al., 1983).

Tumour therapy with monoclonal antibodies has largely been confined to lymphoid tumours since antibodies to lymphocyte cell surface markers of specific stages of differentiation were the first to be developed. However, therapy with a human anti-glioma monoclonal antibody has also been reported (Philips et al., 1982). The results have so far proved variable presumably for some of the reasons defined below but one striking success has been reported in the case of an anti-idiotype antibody raised to the patient's own tumour tissue in a mouse. This may prove to be a special case since the regression of the tumour may be due to feedback through the immune network (Miller et al., 1982). One of the current complexities of assessing the effects of monoclonal antibodies in tumour therapy is the fact that the tumour is usually one related to the cells of the immune system and is being treated by products of other cells of the immune system.

The mechanisms by which such therapy may be effected are not fully resolved but probably involve opsonisation, activation of the complement system and blocking of target cell function (Fig. 1.7). Comparatively few murine antibodies fix human complement but many rat ones are reported to do this (Clark et al., 1983). If a murine antibody is used in human therapy it may also operate by stimulating a host response to the foreign antibody bound to its target cell.

Therapy of this type is not always successful and any remission obtained may be temporary (Fig. 1.8). One reason for this in the case of murine antibodies may obviously be host rejection. However, in addition the cells may undergo antigenic modulation and lose the target antigen. Another possibility is the emergence of an unreactive subpopulation of tumour cells. It is also possible that the antibody will be rendered inactive because it combines with free antigen released from the tumour cells and fails to reach them in consequence (Hamblin et al., 1980; Nadler et al., 1980). A further major problem may simply be access of the antibody to the tumour cell, particularly if the tumour is a solid one or if the antibody is of the IgM class.

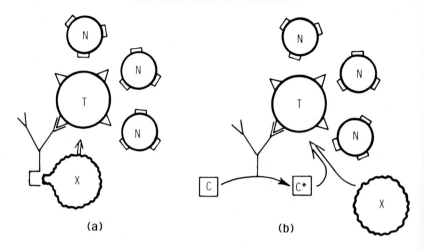

(a)

(b)

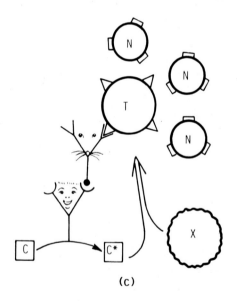

(c)

Much interest has been generated by the observations that, at least in vitro, antibodies may be used to transport toxic materials to the tumour cells while leaving neighbouring normal cells undamaged (Fig. 1.9). These toxic materials may be cytotoxic drugs which may be transported either covalently linked to the antibody (Hurwitz et al., 1975) or in liposomes (Leserman et al., 1981), immunomodulating agents such as interferon, or toxins. In this last case, much interest has been shown in the possible use of ricin or diphtheria toxin covalently linked to the antibody and such systems can be shown to be selectively cytotoxic to a chosen population of cells in mixed cell culture (Krolick et al., 1980; Gilliland et al., 1980; Youle et al., 1980). However, therapy with such powerful reagents is obviously not to be undertaken lightly particularly in light of the unexpected cross-reactivities which can occur with cell surface antigens, all of which would have to be extensively screened (Section 1.2.3).

Human monoclonal antibodies are likely to prove of considerable value in immunosuppression in heart and kidney transplant recipients as well as in the prevention of both graft versus host and host versus graft disease in bone marrow transplantation. Antibodies specifically directed to cytotoxic T cells may have considerable value in these conditions. This type of antibody may also have therapeutic potential in the control of autoimmune disorders. While it may be possible to use murine antibodies for some of these purposes, the length of the period of therapy and amounts of antibody required may preclude the use of a foreign antibody because of the extent of the host rejection of the antibody itself.

Fig. 1.7. Possible mechanisms of antibody mediated tumour cell destruction. (a) A rodent monoclonal antibody binds to a tumour cell (T) associated antigen but not to the normal cells surrounding the tumour (N). Opsonisation leads to the binding of phagocytic cells (X) which can engulf the tumour cell. (b) A rodent monoclonal antibody activates the host complement pathway leading to the attraction of phagocytic cells which engulf the antigen. (c) The host system recognises the rodent antibody as foreign and host antibodies bind to the rodent antibody_tumour cell complex resulting in opsonisation and/or the activation of the host complement system and consequent tumour cell destruction.

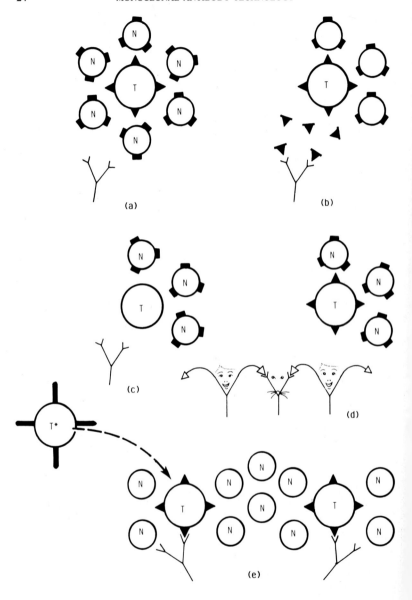

An obvious application of human monoclonal antibodies is in the immunotherapy of rhesus negative mothers. At the moment donors of serum are increasingly hard to obtain and a human monoclonal antibody has been produced by the Epstein Barr virus transformation method. It is currently undergoing clinical trials (Crawford et al., 1983a, b).

Other possible uses of human monoclonal antibodies are in the therapy of viral diseases such as hepatitis and in the treatment of snake venom or other forms of poisoning. In the long term there may be possibilities of specific immune therapy for autoimmune disease such as the use of anti-idiotype antibodies (Fig. 1.10). Alternatively monoclonal antibodies directed to the products of genes controlling the immune response may have therapeutic value. However these applications are little developed at the present though trials on animal systems have been undertaken (Newsome-Davis, 1981; Waldor et al., 1983).

1.3.3. Preparative uses

The earliest most successful preparative use of monoclonal antibodies was in the purification of alpha interferon (Secher and Burke, 1980). In principle, it should be possible to immobilise any monoclonal antibody on an affinity column and use it to obtain large quantities of the required antigen from a crude mixture (Fig. 1.11). To perform such an experiment it should not again in principle be necessary to purify the original immunising antigen though a selection assay must

---

Fig. 1.8. Possible mechanisms to the account for the failure of antibody mediated tumour cell destruction. (a) The antibody has no access to the tumour cell. (b) Dying tumour cells shed antigen which complexes with the free antibody so that it is not available to bind to further tumour cells. (c) The tumour cell no longer has the relevant antigen. Either this has been internalised or a subpopulation of tumour cells without the antigen have been selected. (d) The rodent antibody used in this case is engulfed and destroyed by the host immune response before it reaches the tumour cell. (e) The tumourogenic cell is a minor component of the tumour mass and differentiates to progeny which lack the tumour antigen. Cells bearing the antigen will thus return after initial therapy.

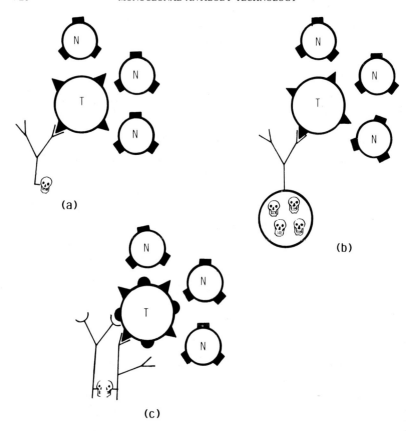

Fig. 1.9. Possible mechanisms of tumour therapy with toxins. (a) The toxin is a drug or poison covalently bound to the antigen. (b) A population of drug molecules is delivered to the vicinity of the tumour cell by an antibody coated liposome. (c) Two synergistic toxins or fragments of toxin are delivered to the tumour cell by antibodies of different type both directed to tumour associated antigens.

Fig. 1.10. Possible mechanisms of anti-idiotype therapy in autoimmune disease. (a) The patient makes antibody 1 to self protein at determinant A. (b) A hybridoma secreting antibody 1 is established by selection with the protein. (c) A hybridoma secreting antibody 2 which reacts with the idiotype of antibody 1 is established by selection with antibody 1. (d) In therapy, antibody 2 reacts with antibody 1 so that it can no longer bind to the self protein at A.

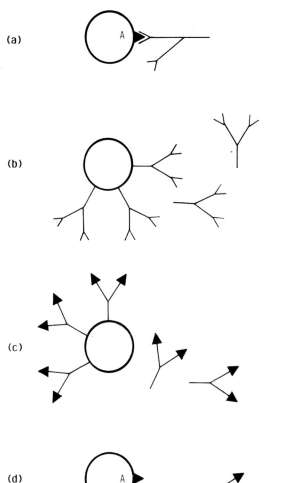

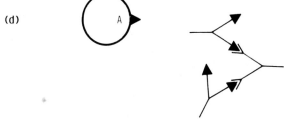

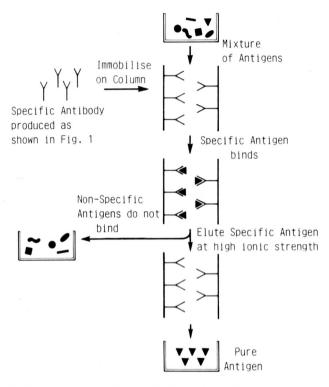

Fig. 1.11. The use of a monoclonal antibody for the purification of a minor antigen in a complex mixture.

be specific for the chosen antigen. In practice this is not always the most effective approach since the major antigens which dominate the serum antibodies also dominate the lymphocyte population used in a cell fusion experiment and if an antibody to a minor antigen is required it is not readily isolated. In theory this problem can be circumvented by performing a sequential series of fusion experiments. In the early ones the antibodies to the major antigens can be isolated and used to remove these antigens from the mixture which is used to immunise subsequent mice so that a large panel of antibodies to minor antigens may be prepared (Fig. 4.1). However, comparatively few of such purification schedules have yet been reported in the literature and it would appear that this procedure is not simple in practice. Other possible ways of handling this problem involve the introduction of more complex immunisation and screening schedules so that the unwanted antibodies are not selected either because tolerance has been induced or the selection procedure is timed to avoid them (for example selection for IgM a short period of time after boosting a mouse extensively preimmunised with the unwanted major antigen).

One undoubted preparative advantage of monoclonal antibodies is the possibility of selection of an antibody of chosen affinity for purification. Where conventional sera are employed, the affinity may be so high as to make recovery of the antigen from the preparative column extremely difficult without the use of extreme denaturing conditions which cause irreversible damage. A monoclonal antibody of submaximal affinity would obviously be of value in such a circumstance (Section 1.2.4).

Preparative uses of monoclonal antibodies are in the early stages as yet in comparison to diagnostic uses. However in the long term they may be of considerable value in many branches of industry.

1.3.4. Basic research

The potential of monoclonal antibodies in basic research is considerable though much less widely discussed than the more immediately obvious applications. In principle they can resolve a single protein from a complex mixture or indeed a single epitope responsible for a specific function of a complex macromolecule. They have already been widely used in basic enzymology, in nucleic acid structural studies, and in the analysis of hormone receptors. It is customary now for any group working on a macromolecule to both clone the genes coding for it and make monoclonal antibodies to it (sometimes without a clear objective for their application). One field of research in which monoclonal antibodies may prove of particular value is in the study of chromosomal proteins. The search for those chromosomal proteins which are responsible for determining cell phenotype has been particularly long and comparatively fruitless and monoclonal antibodies are ideal tools for the dissection of the complex mixture of proteins (Saumweber et al., 1980; Turner, 1981; Hugle et al., 1982; Bhorjee et al., 1983). As hybridoma production becomes a more routine laboratory technique it is likely that this aspect of their application will expand considerably.

1.3.5. T cell hybridomas

The role of the T lymphocyte in the immune response is still poorly understood in comparison to that of the B cell. The response is cellular in that the receptor which recognises the antigen is on the surface of a T lymphocyte. However, it does not recognise the antigen alone but rather the antigen which has been processed by a macrophage or dendritic cell. Individual T cells may have a highly specific response to the antigen, recognising only a small number of, say amino acid residues in the same way as B cell derived antibodies do, and the macrophage in some way processes the antigenic molecule to present these residues on the cell surface. However, an additional complication is that the T cell cannot recognise this small region of antigen alone but must do so in combination with the histocompatibility antigens on the surface of the presenting cell. There is still dispute as to whether the antigen fragment and histocompatibility antigen actually form a composite recognition site, or are recognised separately by two parts of the same receptor (or even different receptors though this is unlikely).

After recognition of the antigen, clonal development of the appropriate cell line occurs. There are many functional subsets of T cells and the T cell progeny thus produced may have a variety of functions and it is clear that T cells are not just a single group but rather a large family of lymphocytes, each of which has a different response still to be understood. Most established T cell lines with known antigen recognition and known functions, secrete lymphokines which attract and activate scavenger cells to the site of the invasion by foreign material. However, some T cells develop cytotoxic functions for cells invaded by intracellular viruses or fungi and other develop helper functions which stimulate B cell antibody production in a manner which is as yet poorly understood (reviewed in most recent immunology textbooks, Section 1.1).

T cell hybridomas are still rare but it is possible to grow T cells from immunised animals in culture for short periods of time and stimulate them with antigen and T cell growth factor (TCGF) (Beezley and Ruddle, 1982; Haas and Von Boehmer, 1982). Alternatively a T cell hybridoma may be made by fusing the lymphoid tissue or the enriched T cell population from the lymphoid tissue of immunised animals with a T cell leukemia partner (analogous to the B cell myeloma lines but derived from a T cell tumour, usually made HAT-sensitive). T cells which respond by expressing some sort of function such as the secretion of a lymphokine may then be cloned by the Fluorescence Activated Cell Sorter (Section 6.3) or tested for loss of function on reaction with both antibodies to the antigen itself and antibodies to the appropriate histocompatibility antigen.

T cell clones isolated in this way have immense potential for both basic and applied research. Firstly, they may be used to isolate the elusive T cell receptor. This is present in such small quantities on the cell surface that large numbers of cells are necessary. This is possible with a T cell hybridoma and the T cells which produce a response such as lymphokine secretion specific to a particular specific antigen and histocompatibility antigen may then be used to immunise a mouse to produce B cell hybridomas. Antibodies secreted by these which block the T cell function are then used to purify the T cell receptor and the handful of experiments of this type which have been performed suggest that this is a heterodimer of molecular weight around 90 000 in both mouse and human systems (e.g. Kappler et al., 1981, 1983). The nature of the dual recognition of both specific and histocompatibility antigens may then be analysed.

Secondly, the B cell antibodies to the T cell receptors may then be used to isolate the RNA coding for these receptors. This will then answer the question of whether recognition of antigen in both systems occurs by the same or by different genes and allow the T cell repertoire to be analysed. This is, to date, one of the major unsolved problems in immunogenetics.

A third contribution of T cell hybridomas to basic research lies in the analysis of the functions of different T cell clones. The differential functions of helper, suppressor, cytotoxic and lymphokine-releasing T cell clones can then be dissected.

The implications of such information for basic research are obvious since it is the T cell response which is thought to be the major contribution to defense against viral infection, tumours and transplantation. It is likely that T cell hybridomas will have immense therapeutic value over the next decade.

The technology of T cell hybridoma production is 4–5 years behind that of B cell hybridoma production but developing fast (see Fathman and Fitch, 1982 and Hammerling et al., 1982 for reviews). Both murine (Kapp et al., 1980) and human (Okada et al., 1981; Foung et al., 1982) T cell hybridomas have been generated and suitable T cell fusion partners are described in Chapter 3. The most recent work is reviewed by Berzofsky (1983).

CHAPTER 2

Assay techniques

2.1. General assay requirements

The assay system is probably the most critical factor in the generation of a large panel of good hybridomas. The emerging clones secrete small amounts of antibody and early cloning of positive samples (Chapter 8) is a key factor in the production of successful clones. This requires a very sensitive assay indeed and many of the assay systems which work well with serum are not of the required level of sensitivity. Additionally, many conventional assays such as those involving immunoprecipitation, depend on multiple epitopes on the antigen and these are ill suited to hybridoma selection.

It is almost impossible to emphasise too often that the final use of the antibody should wherever possible determine the type of assay employed. If the final assay is known to be relatively insensitive, or hard to use for extensive screening then it may be better to perform the initial screen with a sensitive assay and screen the positive samples by the final application assay.

2.2. Theoretical considerations

The kinetics of antibody–antigen interactions are discussed in detail in classical texts (Steward, 1977, 1978). Most of the earlier antibody kinetic studies were described by the kinetics of a univalent antigen (usually a hapten) and divalent antibody. However, many assay systems have the additional complication of one or other component (usually the antigen) being fixed on a solid phase. Like all reactions between proteins they are dependent on the concentration of both reactants and the conditions under which the reaction takes place. In the case of monoclonal antibody assay these are all highly relevant and may be very different from conventional antibody work. A comprehensive understanding of the theoretical background is essential for the production of a large number of hybridomas secreting antibody of the required characteristics. The subject is introduced in Section 1.2.4.

2.2.1. Rate of association

The initial rate of association of an antibody with an antigen is described by the classic equation:

Rate of formation of product $= K_1$ (antibody) (antigen)

In this context, monoclonal antibodies are very different indeed from polyclonal ones. The number of epitopes on the antigen is much reduced and in the case of a small protein is usually only one. Thus the effective concentration of the antigen is very low. The antibody will still be bivalent (or decavalent in the case of an IgM) but its concentration may be very low. This is particularly true in the case of early assay (which is advisable in order to detect suitable clones in order to avoid overgrowth by revertants which have lost the appropriate chromosomes). Additionally, however, clones vary greatly in the amount of antibody that they are able to secrete and human clones in particular are likely to secrete very small amounts of specific antibody (Chapter 3). In these circumstances therefore the concentration of effective antibody is likely to be exceptionally low. As a consequence of this, the parameters on the right-hand side of the equation defining the association rate are liable to be several orders of magnitude below those in conventional serum and indeed below those in the serum of the mouse, rat or human used in the testing of the chosen assay. As a result, the conventional assay time of periods of one or two hours at room temperature or 37 °C have very limited relevance. A longer incubation time of antibody or antigen during screening may lead to the detection of several clones which could otherwise be regarded as negative (see, however, Section 2.6 if an ELISA assay is to be used as antigen may leach from the plates if a long assay time is employed). The association rate is usually the parameter which determines the final equilibrium constant (see Section 2.2.3) and the concentration of antigen in most assays remains constant. However, by assaying for too short a time, or too early when the antibody concentration is low, it is possible to miss an antibody which may be suitable for the required purpose but is secreted in small amounts at early stages or an antibody which is suitable for the required purpose but which is of comparatively low affinity.

The situation defined above is altered by the fact that most antibodies are at least divalent. However, for most assays at initial stages where antibody and antigen concentration are low they may be regarded as univalent. The antigen may also be multivalent as in cell or bacterial surface epitopes. These are covered in Section 2.2.4.

2.2.2. Rate of dissociation

The dissociation rate of an antibody antigen complex is defined by the equation:

$$\text{Initial rate of dissociation} = K_2 \text{ (antibody–antigen)}$$

With most antibody–antigen reactions, it is the dissociation rate rather than the association rate that determines the affinity as the dissociation rate can vary over 8–9 orders of magnitude but is nearly always very much lower than the association rate. Additionally, with conventional reactions there are many complexes formed between different antibodies and their epitopes so that, at any one time, there is still substantial reaction towards complex formation. The dissociation rate is not only the most variable among different antibodies under a defined set of conditions but also the most variable in a single antibody with respect to environmental conditions such as pH, temperature, etc. (Mason and Williams, 1980). The forward reaction in the three antibodies described by Mason and Williams shows only small variations with respect to temperature but the dissociation reaction shows differences in orders of magnitude. While this sample is small, it suggests that for the antigens described, assay at *lower* temperatures is more likely to detect positive samples after an over-night period at 4 °C than assays for the same time at higher tempera-tures, especially if the antibody concentration is low.

2.2.3. Equilibrium concentration of reactants

The equilibrium constant for an antibody antigen reaction is the ratio of the forward to the backward rates

i.e. $K_{eq} = K_1/K_2$

or $K_{eq} = (Ab-Ag)/(Ab)(Ag)$

Thus the equilibrium situation, which is the most suitable for assay, is dependent on the ratios of the considerations in Sections 2.2.1 and 2.2.2. From these it is clear that the concentrations of the reactants and the assay conditions may influence the possibility of detection of a suitable hybridoma. Thus with polyclonal sera it is usually consider-ed reasonable to assume that an optimal equilibrium condition will be achieved by incubation for an hour or two at room temperature, and biological pH, ionic strength, etc. Monoclonal antibodies at early screening may not be detected unless several of these parameters are varied and it seems more than likely that antibodies to more interest-ing or relevant epitopes will be detected when it becomes possible to extend screening procedures to cover a variety of parameters.

2.2.4. Effect of multivalence

All antibodies are at least divalent and IgA and IgM antibodies may have several idiotypes on the same molecule. Additionally, many antigens have neighbouring epitopes. Multivalent antibodies are usu-ally helpful to screening procedures since the effective dissociation rate can be reduced if enough antigen is present. If one antibody-com-bining region dissociates from the antigen, the chances of it or its partner reassociating are increased because of their geometric proxim-ity. It is possible that assay selection procedures alone account for the relatively high numbers of IgM secreting hybridomas produced in many fusions.

If the antigen has a large number of epitopes then this can affect the reaction in several ways. Antigens with multiple epitopes are probably most commonly encountered in bacterial systems with symmetrical cell wall structures. They can also occur in situations in which large amounts of antigen have been bound to a solid surface. If the antibody is in excess in such a system it may bind through only one of its possibly variable regions and consequently it may dissociate more readily than an antibody with two regions anchored. Consequently there are rare situations in which an ELISA assay for example may detect antibodies better if small amounts of material are bound to each well.

2.2.5. Specificity and affinity

The complex relationship between specificity and affinity is discussed in Section 1.2.6. Much of this information is based on a paper by Mossman et al. (1980) who showed that monoclonal antibodies against polymorphic antigens could exhibit extreme specificity in one type of assay and considerable epitope overlap in a second higher affinity assay. Nonetheless, it is assumed that at least in the initial stages, an assay detecting the maximum numbers of positive clones is required. Suitable conditions for obtaining specific responses can then be achieved at a later stage.

2.3. Practical considerations

2.3.1. Numbers of assays

The number of plates to be used in the initial fusions and in subsequent clonings is discussed in Chapter 6 and 8. In a typical fusion procedure utilising 4 × 96 well plates some 400 samples must be assayed in a short period of time. Subcloning usually involves a similar number although a valuable clone may be subcloned with more. Additionally, as discussed in Section 2.2, a comprehensive screen of hybridomas should ideally involve the use of several plates under different sets of assay conditions. With mouse systems it is exceptionally valuable to assay as early as possible in order to decide which cells should be cloned before overgrowth by non-secretors occurs. With rat systems this is less essential and with human ones there is not enough data on established hybridomas to delineate a clear production pathway but the antibody concentration is likely to be low and consequently screening should be comprehensive and also performed more than once (i.e. early to detect high affinity/high producing clones and later to detect lower affinity or lower yield clones). The number of assays involved is consequently considerable and individual screening by, say, immunocytochemical techniques, is likely to be either impractical or inevitably less comprehensive. To cope with the numbers a broad screening system which can be easily handled is recommended. If this system is far removed from the final application of the antibody then positive samples detected by the first screen should be assayed by a second directed to the final application, since the number of positives is very much lower than the total number of clones.

2.3.2. Time of assay

In terms of clonal growth the time of assay should be soon after clones are microscopically visible and again a few days after when clones are visible to the eye (Sections 2.2 and 2.3 above). Screening should continue for several weeks.

The time of the actual assay procedure is a different consideration influenced very much by the antibody concentration as discussed in Section 2.2.

However, it should ideally be for a very much longer period than the conventional serum from the mouse used for fusion to allow for the low antibody concentration as discussed in Section 2.2.1. Where a solid phase ELISA utilising non-convalently bound antigen is employed, this requirement must be balanced against the tendency of the antigen to leach from the plate (Lehtonen and Viljonen, 1980a).

2.3.3. pH of assay

It may be expected that most antibodies will have their optimal reaction with antigen at physiological pH. At least in some cases (Mossman et al., 1980; Fraser et al., 1982; Fig. 2.1) this is not accurate nor would it be expected to be so from a consideration of the essentially random nature of antibody diversity (Tonegawa, 1983). It is quite possible to fail to detect a good hybridoma by screening at a single pH. However if the final use of the antibody must be at a certain pH value, there is no point in screening at other pH values.

The pH of tissue culture fluid in which cells are growing can vary over almost a whole pH unit. Spent medium from rapidly growing

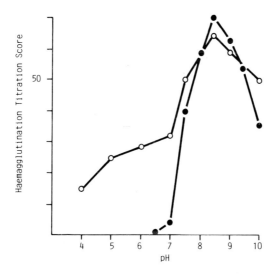

Fig. 2.1. pH dependence of a monoclonal antibody directed to the human N blood group antigen in comparison to serum antibody. The serum antibody can be detected at most pH values but the monoclonal is not detectable by this assay below pH 7. •, monoclonal antibody; o, serum. (Courtesy of Dr. Robin Fraser and Dr. Angus Munro.)

cells can be well below pH 7. Most assay procedures involve direct transfer of material from the tissue culture wells to the assay plates and thus in any screening procedure, pH becomes a natural variable. Polyclonal sera usually react over a wide range but monoclonal antibodies may have very defined and discrete optima. If a defined pH is required for the final application then the assay should be buffered accordingly during the incubation of antibody with antigen. This may be particularly relevant for in vivo uses.

Where pH adjustments are necessary the nature of the buffer should also be considered as the buffer components themselves may affect the assay (i.e. phosphate buffers with nucleic acid antigens).

2.3.4. Temperature of assay

It has already been mentioned in Section 2.2 that the dissociation constant is the variable which is most sensitive to temperature and consequently this parameter should be varied if two assays of the same supernatant are possible. The current limited evidence suggests that the best assay conditions for hybridomas favour incubation at 4° rather than at room temperature or higher but ideally both should be attempted unless the final use precludes a certain temperature.

2.3.5. Ionic strength of assay

There is no detailed information available on the ionic strength variations in hybridoma assays. However, since a protein–protein interaction is involved, it seems likely that the usual considerations apply. Non-specific binding is more likely to occur at low ionic strengths. If pH variations are used in the assay then all the buffers used should have the same ionic strength.

2.4. Antibody sampling

It has been emphasised in Section 2.2 that the amount of antibody available in the supernatant of a newly established hybridoma is small. Antibodies, like other proteins, will be adsorbed readily on surfaces of glass or synthetic materials. The albumin (and possibly the small amount of γ-globulin) in the fetal calf serum should minimise this, blocking most sites. However, albumin is a less than ideal blocking reagent since its isoelectric point is several units of pH above that of γ-globulins and it is possible that albumin does not therefore occupy all possible blocking sites on sampling material.

Any assay system which involves multiple transfers of the antibody from the tissue culture plate to the final assay is therefore not only cumbersome and inconvenient but unwise since antibody may be lost on surfaces. Equipment used for transfer should be pre-treated with bovine γ-globulin or serum in order to minimise this. In addition, many sampling devices which allow more convenient transfer or even direct assay are now marketed (e.g. Dynatech). If these devices are to be immersed in the tissue culture plate, they must, of course, be sterilised as well as blocked. It is also possible to assay using short term tissue culture of hybridomas in antigen coated plates and thus avoid any transfers at all (Weetman et al., 1982).

2.5. Types of assay

It is difficult to classify the possible types of assay for hybridomas without consideration of the relevant antigen. However, the fact that the assay should ideally be as close as possible to the final use of the monoclonal antibody cannot be overemphasised. The condition of the antigen (formaldehyde fixed, radiolabelled, bound to other molecules, accessible or inaccessible in cells) should be as similar as possible in the screening assay as in the final use. The assay conditions (Sections 2.2 and 2.3) should also be similar. Historically, cellular assays were the first to be used for hybridoma detection (Kohler and Milstein, 1975). In more recent years solid-phase assay systems have become by far the most common. However, liquid-phase assays such as radioimmunoassay are also frequently used. Biological assays are the least common. Solid-phase assays are covered in the greatest detail in this text as they are sensitive, readily adaptable to a large number of antigens, economical, and easy to perform on a large number of samples.

2.6. Solid-phase assays

The solid-phase assay system is adaptable to almost any antigen with almost any antibody. Its development is comparatively recent and the growth of the use of ELISA (Enzyme Linked Immuno Sorbent Assay) assays in particular has been logarithmic since the first reported use by Engvall and Perlman in 1971 (reviewed in Engvall and Pesce, 1982). Two major types of assay are shown in Figs. 2.2 and 2.3. In the ELISA or radioactive binding assay the antigen is bound to the plate and incubated with the monoclonal antibody. A second antibody coupled to an enzyme or isotope is then used to detect the first. In the sandwich or IRMA (Immuno Radio-Metric Assay) assay one antibody which may or may not be monoclonal is bound to the solid

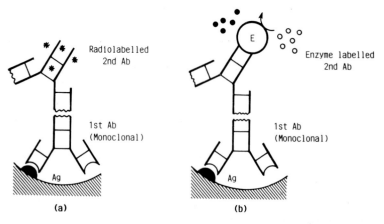

Fig. 2.2. Solid-phase binding assays for specific antibody. (a) Solid-phase binding of radioactive second antibody (sometimes referred to as RIA). (b) Solid-phase binding of enzyme-labelled second antibody (ELISA). o, substrate; •, coloured product.

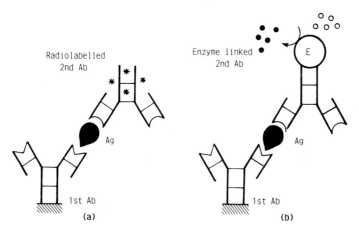

Fig. 2.3. Solid-phase binding assays for specific antigen (IRMA). (a) The radio-labell-
ed second antibody is directed to a different epitope from that used by the first antibody
bound to the plate. (b) The enzyme-linked second antibody is directed to a different
epitope from the plate bound first antibody.

support, the antigen is then added, and a second labelled antibody
directed towards a different epitope on the antigen is used to detect
the bound antigen. The first system is generally used for screening and
quantitating antibody and the second one for quantitating antigen.
However, if both antibodies are of different species, the second assay
may be adapted for screening with the use of a third labelled anti-
species antibody. In principle, many types of sandwich assay with
increasing layers may be developed but each additional layer adds to
the uncertainty of the assay, to the complexity of performing it, and
to the risk of antigen leaking from the solid support. Solid-phase
assays of both types can be adapted for the use of small molecules
by haptenisation.

2.6.1. The nature of the solid support

The chemical nature of the solid support may be glass (Engvall and
Perlman, 1971), nylon (Hendry and Herrman, 1980), sepharose,

cellulose (Giallongo et al., 1982; King and Kochoumian, 1979), cyanogen bromide or DBM activated paper (Lehtonen and Viljanen, 1980; Locker and Motta, 1983), or nitrocellulose paper (Hawkes et al., 1982; Smith et al., 1984). However, the most common are polyvinyl or polystyrene. The physical nature can be balls (Ziola et al., 1977), rings (Lehtonen and Viljanen, 1980a), beads of varying capacity (Giallongo et al., 1982; Hendry and Herrman, 1980), and discs or sheets of paper. However, the great majority of assays are performed with a solid phase support which is in the form of a 96-well polystyrene or polyvinyl plate. The plates are generally coated with material which encourages the binding of the antigen. Manufacturers are usually elusive about the actual constitution of the plate and the coating material and use names such as 'Immunolon' which are uninformative. This type of plate is marketed by all the major manufacturers (Flow, Gibco, Biorad, Dynatech) and the performance may vary widely under assay conditions. Some give good positives with sera from immunised animals but also a high background with negative serum and in any preliminary test of plates it is the signal to noise ratio rather than the signal strength which should be evaluated. While it has been emphasised that maximum sensitivity is necessary for early screening the plates contribute substantially to the cost of hybridoma production and more economical ones of slightly lower sensitivity are frequently employed. To test the suitability of plates it is advisable to obtain a small batch of each and test with controls with and without antigen and with positive and negative serum to ascertain both the background and the strength of the signal for each type of plate. Another good test of plate quality is the ability of results to duplicate between two plates and between two wells in the same plate. Experience in our own laboratory to date with a wide variety of antigens suggests that at the moment, the cost reflects the quality of the plates but this may change. There is no point in accepting manufacturers figures for an antigen or antiserum not identical to the ones being used for hybridoma production.

Although microtitre plates made of polyvinyl or polystyrene are the most common support, consideration should be given to the use of nitrocellulose or other types of paper support (Hawkes et al., 1982) as they are exceptionally easy and economical to use.

2.6.2. Attachment of antigen

Most soluble protein and nucleic acid antigens are passively adsorbed onto the solid surface. The capacity of the various supports varies widely. In addition, the amount adsorbed will depend on the diffusion coefficient of the protein, the surface area to volume ratio and the time and temperature of the adsorption incubation. If the antigen is a soluble protein then the microtitre plate is usually coated with 100 µl of a solution of 1–10 µg/ml. More protein can be bound but the percentage bound falls as higher concentrations of protein are used. It must be remembered that the binding is non-covalent and in most systems protein will leach off the plate during subsequent incubation with antibody.

This leaching of antigen may be considerable at high concentrations. It is reported to be in the order of 30% if large amounts are used. Leaching is a fast process and most occurs early in incubation. Nylon supports appear to leak more than polystyrene ones and there is limited evidence to suggest that polyvinyl supports may leach less dramatically (Frankel and Herhard, 1979). In theory such levels of leaching could have serious consequences, not because there is not enough antigen remaining bound to perform the assay, but rather because the unbound antigen can complex the monoclonal antibody thus reducing its binding. However, most experiments to test leaching have been carried out at comparatively high antigen densities and it is likely that leaching is less serious at low antigen densities. Antigen density variations can affect not only the sensitivity of the assay but the affinity of the monoclonal antibody selected in this way (Lehtonen and Viljanen, 1980b; Pesce et al., 1978; Bruins et al., 1978).

Consequently, there is no particular advantage to be gained from binding a large amount of antigen to the solid support and there may be disadvantages in binding too much. However, too much washing or long periods of washing are to be avoided. Early ELISA assays suggested that the antigen bound better at high pH values. However, since the subsequent washes and incubations are usually at physiological pH values this is probably unnecessary and potentially damaging to a screening process of an antigen bound at a high pH which may leach more readily at physiological pH thus preventing the binding of the monoclonal antibody.

Binding a protein to a solid phase denatures it to some extent as shown by loss of enzymatic activity (Berkowitz and Webert, 1981). Where immunological activity is relevant this may lead to the selection of monoclonal antibodies which bind to epitopes not available in the native protein. Consequently it is sometimes possible for antibodies to be selected by a solid phase binding assay and found unreactive in a liquid-phase assay (Miller et al., 1983).

Many solid-phase assays are now performed with particulate material such as chromosomes, viruses, bacteria, parasites or whole cells. While the smaller among these may occasionally be effectively absorbed onto plates in the same manner as soluble proteins (MacCormack et al., 1982) it is usual for the larger antigens and in particular whole cells, to be fixed in some way to the plate. This is most commonly performed with the use of 10–50 µg/ml poly-L-lysine to precoat the plate for an hour at room temperatures. The excess polylysine is removed and the cells are then added in 100 µl of buffer at a concentration of between 5×10^3 and 5×10^4/ml for 45–60 min. The cells may then be fixed with glutaraldehyde (0.1–0.25%) for 3–5 min and washed thoroughly. After blocking of the reactive sites (Section 2.6.3) the coated plates may be stored (see Section 2.6.4) for several weeks without loss of immunoactivity (Heusser et al., 1981; Suter et al., 1980). Glutaraldehyde may destroy some of the antigenic determinants but the evidence suggests that at the concentrations involved this effect is not appreciable. However, unfixed cells may also be assayed by pre-blocking of the microtitre plate and centrifugation of the cells at each stage (Section 2.8).

Other methods of fixation of cells such as vacuum desiccation have also been reported (Douillard et al., 1980). A method for coupling bacterial polysaccharide antigens has also been published (Gray, 1979).

2.6.3. Blocking of remaining sites on the solid support

Most solid supports adsorb proteins non-specifically by hydrophobic interactions as discussed in Section 2.6.1. It is evident that they will also adsorb the antibody if the plates are not fully saturated with antigen. Once the antigen has been bound it is therefore usual to block any other sites on the support by the use of bovine serum albumin (typically at 1% w/v), gelatin (0.2–0.5% w/v), non-specific serum (typically at 1% v/v) or bovine γ-globulin (1% w/v) dissolved in phosphate-buffered saline. The last two are probably better as they contain irrelevant antibodies which conform more closely to the charge and size of the specific antibody. However, they should not be employed if Protein A is being used in the detection system (Section 9.7.2). The use of 0.01% Tween 20 or Triton X-100 in subsequent buffers also reduces the background as it discourages the formation of further hydrophobic interactions between the solid support and first and second antibodies. Additionally, if glutaraldehyde has been used, it is advisable to wash the plates with 100 mM glycine in the buffer to block off any remaining reactive glutaraldehyde sites.

2.6.4. Storage of antigen-bound solid supports

Most antigen bound microtitre plates can be stored at 4 °C for several weeks. 0.02% sodium azide is incubated with the blocking buffer to avoid bacterial contamination and the plates are stored with blocking buffer present to avoid antigen desorption. This is washed off immediately before use. If the second antibody is labelled with peroxidase it should be noted that azide inhibits this and must be removed in the washing. Dried antigen bound to nitrocellulose paper may also be stored for long periods (Smith et al., 1984).

2.6.5. Incubation with antigen

Many of the problems associated in the incubation with the antigen have already been discussed in detail in Sections 2.2 and 2.3. In particular, it is desirable to have an assay which allows fairly long periods of incubations with the monoclonal antibody so that small amounts may be detected. In a solid-phase assay, this has to balance against the tendency of the antigen to leach off the plate during the incubation (Section 2.6.1). The extent of this can be monitored by performing the original chequerboard assay (Fig. 2.4) with duplicate plates incubated for different periods of time (overnight at 4 °C and 2 h at room temperature) with the antiserum from the immunised animal. With polyclonal antiserum the effects of low antigen concentration discussed in Section 2.2 are likely to be very much less pronounced and leaching is likely to be the more relevant contributory factor to variation. It is possible to incubate antigen coated plates with the hybridoma cells themselves in short term tissue culture (Weetman et al., 1982).

2.6.6. The nature of the second antibody

The bound monoclonal antibody is usually detected with a second antibody directed against it. Covalently linked to this second antibody can be an enzyme with a chromogenic substrate. Sheep anti mouse or goat anti mouse enzyme antibodies linked to enzyme are thus used to detect murine hybridomas. Alternatively, radiolabelled second antibody may be used although this has become less common for screening. Enzyme-linked second antibodies are available from a large number of commercial companies (Miles, Flow, Sigma, Bio-Rad, etc.) and the quality is highly variable. Radioiodine-labelled second antibodies are usually made in the laboratory by one of the several methods used to attach iodine to proteins (Johnstone and Thorpe, 1982). While Protein A has been used to screen for monoclonal antibodies it is in general an unreliable reagent because of the considerable variation in binding among and within classes of IgG (Section

9.7) and the failure of Protein A to bind to IgM. It is, however, an excellent reagent if used against polyclonal rabbit antisera and so it is possible to use rabbit sera directed against the species in which the hybridoma has been raised and to follow this with enzyme or radiolabelled protein A.

The second antibody itself is usually directed against the total IgG of the species in which the hybridoma is being produced. Most commercially available second antibodies linked to enzymes are not affinity purified although some are. An IgM, IgA or IgE monoclonal antibody will be detected by this reagent because it will react with determinants on the light chains, but the signal may be lowered because of the smaller number of overall epitopes so that a hybridoma secreting large amount of antibody of a class other than IgG may appear only weakly positive on screening (Fig. 2.4). Enzyme-linked second antibodies directed specifically to heavy chain epitopes may also be obtained. These can be used where a specific class of antibody is required but are in general more expensive.

2.6.7. Enzymes used in ELISA

There are three enzymes generally used for colour development with the second antibody. The earliest was alkaline phosphatase (usually from calf intestine) and the commonest now is horseradish peroxidase. The third is β-galactosidase from *E. coli* which is active at the higher pH values preferred for antigen adsorption. Phosphatase or galactosidase are used in situations where there may be endogenous peroxidase activity in the antigen. However, there are several other enzymes occasionally used since the detection system only requires that the enzyme have a chromogenic substrate and any enzyme which releases a hydrogen or hydroxyl ion can be used in conjunction with a pH indicator. Conjugation is by a variety of methods, the commonest being glutaraldehyde (O'Sullivan and Marks, 1981). Conjugation inevitably involves loss of activity to some extent and Milstein and Cuello (1983) have developed bifunctional antibodies to minimise this. Other reagents involving the more specific linkage of antibody to enzyme by disulphide bonds have been suggested to give better specific activity (King and Kochoumian, 1979). Commercial preparation of any of the three enzymes linked to a second antibody vary widely in quality depending on the specificity of the antibody, the specific activity of the enzyme, and the methodology of covalent linking.

The substrates generally employed for alkaline phosphatase and β-galactosidase are p-nitrophenylphosphate and o-nitrophenyl β-D-galactopyranoside respectively with colour development being detected at 405 and 420 nm. In the case of horseradish peroxidase several substrates are marketed although o-phenylenediamine (OPD) is most commonly used. This is mildly carcinogenic and claims have been made that non-carcinogenic substrates are as good at detecting the signal. However, Al-Kaissi and Mostratos (1983) have compared several peroxidase substrates and found that the main group of mildly carcinogenic ones are of good quality, OPD being the best and in general better than the non-carcinogenic 5-aminosalicylic acid. Peroxidase assays on paper can be made using conventional substrates if discs are employed but for whole sheets of dot bound antigen (Section 2.6.10) an insoluble product is obviously required so substrates such as 4-chloro-1-naphthol (Smith et al., 1984) are employed.

In conventional immunoassays the peroxidase anti-peroxidase system of second antibody is sometimes preferred. In this system the second antibody is unlabelled and used in excess so that some antibody sites are available to react with a third antibody which is itself an antibody linked to its peroxidase antigen. There is little advantage in using this system for hybridoma screening as it involves extra complex steps. A mouse monoclonal anti-peroxidase hybridoma has been made and is available (Ziegler et al., 1979) but is of no greater sensitivity than the simple peroxidase assay in the experience of the home laboratory.

More sensitive ELISA detection systems may be obtained by the use of fluorogenic substrates for alkaline phosphatase or β-galactosidase (Shalev et al., 1980; Labrousse et al., 1982). An ingenious assay utilising glutamate decarboxylase with a radioactive substrate has also been reported (Fields et al., 1981). However it seems unlikely that such complex assays will find wide applications in hybridoma screening despite their sensitivity.

2.6.8. Detection of signal

Most ELISA assays are read in spectrophotometer adapted for microtitre plates such as the Titretrek Multiscan (Dynatech). This is an excellent method for obtaining printed results for storage and removes the subjective element. It is a comparatively expensive piece of equipment, however, and it is usually possible to judge positive samples by eye. Where the antigen has been bound to a paper support, direct staining of the paper with chloronaphthol leads to a paper sheet with a permanent record (Smith et al., 1983).

Where a radiolabelled second antibody is used it is possible (and necessary if the antigen has been labelled with a beta-emitting isotope) to cut through the plates with a fine wire and count each well (Tsu and Herzenberg, 1980). However, it is usually more convenient to use an iodine-labelled second antibody and autoradiograph the plate.

2.6.9. The chequerboard ELISA for determining optimum conditions of assay

The chequerboard ELISA (Fig. 2.4) is a useful initial test of the assay system when the serum of the animal to be used in the fusion is tested against the antigen which has been used for immunisation. It allows the optimum conditions of antigen coating to be determined, determines the titre of the serum, and checks that all the assay controls are negative. The assay is then readily adapted to a screening one with minimal alterations.

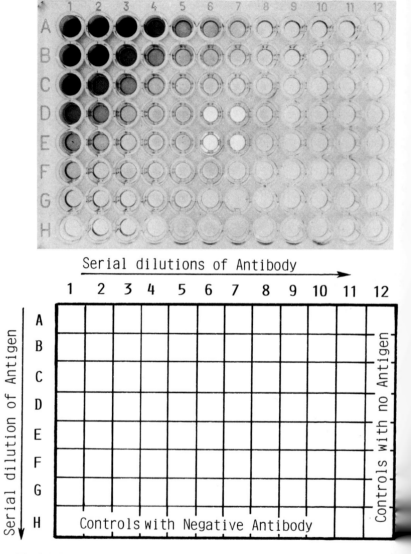

Fig. 2.4. ELISA chequerboard assay. Top, typical results. Bottom, assay design.

Protocol 2.1

Chequerboard ELISA for soluble antigens

(i) Immunise a rat or mouse with antigen (Chapter 5). Boost 4–7 days before bleeding but not killing the animal. Withdraw 0.1–0.2 ml blood (Appendix 1), centrifuge and store serum. Prepare stock negative serum from an unimmunised mouse of the same strain and age.

(ii) Prepare 2.4 ml of antigen in phosphate-buffered saline at approximately 50 µg/ml. Perform a series of 6 doubling dilutions in small tubes so that the final concentration is 1/64 of the starting one and there is 1.2 ml of each sample.

(iii) On a 96-well microtitre plate (Dynatech), pipette 100 µl of the most concentrated antigen solution into all 12 wells of row A, 100 µl of the first dilution into all 12 wells of row B and so on until row G. Put 100 µl of PBS into all 12 wells of row H. Incubate overnight at 4 °C.

(iv) Make up 0.8-ml aliquots of doubling dilutions of the rat or mouse serum starting with 1.6 ml of a 1 in 100 dilution in phosphate-buffered saline containing 0.5 mg/ml BSA and making 10 further dilutions so that the last tube has a 1 in 10 000 dilution of antibody. Make up 1.2 ml of negative serum diluted to 1 in 100 in the same buffer.

(v) Flick or shake the antigen solution from the plate with a sharp wrist movement. Wash the plate once by immersion in coating buffer followed by sharp shaking over a sink to empty all the wells. 'Knock' the plates dry by hammering them face down on wads of paper or cloth towels.

(vi) Incubate the plates for 1 h at room temperature with 100 µl of a solution of 10 mg/ml BSA or 1% bovine serum in coating buffer.

Wash the plates three times with phosphate-buffered saline containing 0.05% Tween 20. Knock dry.

(vii) To each well in column 1 add 100 µl of the 1/100 dilution of antiserum. To each in column 2 add 100 µl of the 1 in 200 and so on. In column 12 add a 1 in 100 dilution of the negative serum. Incubate at room temperature for 1–2 h. Wash three times in phosphate-buffered saline containing 0.05% Tween 20 and knock the plates dry.

(viii) Add 100 μl of horseradish peroxidase anti-mouse (or rat) IgG conjugate (Miles) diluted 1 in 500 with 0.5 mg/ml BSA 0.05% Tween 20. Incubate for 2 h at room temperature. Wash three times in

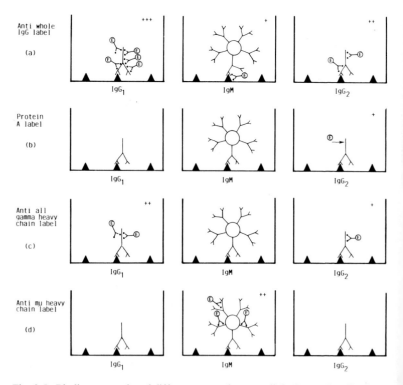

Fig. 2.5. Binding properties of different types of enzyme-linked second antibodies to mouse antibodies. (a) An anti IgG (H + L chain) antibody. This will react with all immunoglobulins because of the light chain specificity. However, most commercial preparations are raised to whole IgG and will consequently favour IgG_1 which is present in larger amounts. (b) Protein A will only react with certain types of IgG depending on the species and not IgM in any species (see Chapter 9). (c) An anti-all IgG heavy chain label classes other than IgG but may still be biased to IgG_1 because it is the predominant antibody used for the production of the detecting antiserum. (d) An antibody directed against the μ heavy chain will only detect IgM secreting hybridomas.

phosphate-buffered saline containing 0.05% Tween 20 and knock the plates dry.

(ix) Add 100 µl of a solution of 0.04 mg/ml of freshly prepared *o*-phenylenediamine (Sigma) dissolved in 0.05 M sodium citrate 0.15 M sodium phosphate pH 6 containing 0.32 µl/ml H_2O_2 (0.01 %). Cover the plate with foil and incubate at room temperature for 30 min. Add 50 µl of 4 N sulphuric acid to stop the reaction. If a multiscanning spectrophotometer is available read the absorbance at 492 nm. Otherwise inspect the plate. The colour is stable for several hours.

Note. If alkaline phosphatase is the preferred enzyme conjugate for use in step (viii) then for step (ix) the substrate solution should be 1 mg/ml *p*-nitrophenylphosphate freshly dissolved in 9.7% v/v diethanolamine buffer pH 9.8. The reaction is stopped by the addition of 50 µl 3 N NaOH. Absorption should be read at 405 nm.

If β-galactosidase is the preferred enzyme conjugate then for step (ix) the substrate solution should be 1 mg/ml *o*-nitrophenyl-β-D-galactopyranoside (Sigma) dissolved in 0.1 M sodium borate, 0.08 M NaCl, 10 mM $MgCl_2$ pH 8.5. The reaction is stopped with 50 µl 1 M Na_2CO_3 and the colour is read at 420 nm.

Protocol 2.2

Chequerboard ELISA for cellular antigens

(i) Immunise a rat or mouse with cellular antigen (Chapter 5). Boost four days before bleeding but not killing the animal. Withdraw 0.1–0.2 ml blood (Appendix 1), centrifuge and store the serum. Prepare stock negative serum from an unimmunised mouse of the same strain and age.

(ii) Dissolve poly-L-lysine (Sigma) in phosphate-buffered saline at a concentration of 10 µg/ml. Dispense 100 µl onto each well of a 96-well microtitre ELISA plate (Dynatech) and incubate at room temperature for 2 h. Flick or shake the solution from the 96-well plate and wash twice by immersion in phosphate-buffered saline followed by sharp shaking. Prepare 2.4 ml of the cellular antigen at 5×10^6 cells/ml. Check microscopically that there is little cell debris. Perform a series of six doubling dilutions in small eppendorf tubes so that the lowest cell density is 7.5×10^4 cells/ml. Pipette 100 µl of the highest cell density into each well in row A, then 100 µl of the next cell density into each well in row B and so on. To row H add 100 µl phosphate-buffered saline. Incubate for 45 min at room temperature and wash the plates in phosphate-buffered saline. Immerse in 0.25% glutaraldehyde for 3 min and wash the plates three times in phosphate-buffered saline. Dry by shaking and knocking dry on wads of paper or cloth towels. Incubate the plates overnight at 4° with 100 µl of 10 mg/ml BSA or 1% bovine serum in PBS containing 0.02% sodium azide and 100 mM glycine. The plates may be stored in this manner.

(iii) Make up 0.8-ml aliquots of doubling dilutions of the rat or mouse serum starting with 1.6 ml of a 1 in 100 dilution in phosphate-buffered saline containing 0.5 mg/ml BSA, then make 10 further dilutions so that the last tube has a 1 in 1000 dilution of antibody. Make up 0.8 ml of negative serum diluted 1 in 100 in the same buffer.

(iv) Wash the plate three times with phosphate-buffered saline containing 0.05% Tween 20. Knock dry.

(v) To each well in column 1 add 100 µl of the 1 in 100 dilutions of the antiserum. To each in column 2 add 100 µl of the 1 in 200 dilution and so on. In column 12 add a 1 in 100 dilution of negative serum. Incubate for 1–2 h at room temperature, wash three times in phosphate-buffered saline, 0.05% Tween 20 and knock dry.

(vi) Add 100 µl of horseradish peroxidase linked anti mouse (or rat) IgG (Miles Laboratories) diluted 1 in 100 with phosphate-buffered saline containing 0.5 mg/ml bovine serum albumin and 0.05% Tween 20. Incubate for 2 h at room temperature, wash three times with phosphate-buffered saline containing 0.05% Tween 20 and knock the plates dry.

(vii) Add 100 µl of a solution of 0.04 mg/ml of freshly prepared o-phenylenediamine dissolved in 0.05 M sodium citrate 0.15 M sodium phosphate pH 6 containing 0.32 µl/ml H_2O_2 (0.01 %). Cover the plate with foil and incubate at room temperature for 30 min. Add 50 µl of 4 N sulphuric acid to stop the reaction. If a multiscanning spectrophotometer is available read the absorbance at 492 nm. Otherwise inspect the plate. The colour is stable for several hours.

Note. If alkaline phosphatase is the preferred enzyme antibody conjugate for use in step (vi) then for step (vi) the substrate solution should be 1 mg/ml *p*-nitrophenylphosphate freshly dissolved in 9.7% v/v diethanolamine buffer pH 9.8. The reaction is stopped by the addition of 50 µl 3 N NaOH. Absorption should be read at 405 nm.

If β-galactosidase is the preferred enzyme antibody conjugate then for step (ix) the substrate solution should be 1 mg/ml *o*-nitrophenyl-β-D-galactopyranoside (Sigma) dissolved in 0.1 M sodium borate, 0.08 M NaCl, 10 mM $MgCl_2$, pH 8.5. The reaction is stopped with 50 µl 1 M Na_2CO_3 and the colour is read at 420 nm.

The appearance of the ELISA plate should be with strong colour in the top left hand corner, fading to weaker colour in the bottom left hand corner. Row (Fig. 2.5) H and column 12 should have very little colour and provide the background. The titre of the animal is estimated by finding the highest dilution at which its serum gives more colour than the negative serum and the wells without antigen. The lowest antigen concentration at which this titre is still observed can then be selected. Potential difficulties in the assay should immediately become apparent by inspection of the controls. The use of a 1 in 100 dilution of negative serum as antibody control is not ideal and a separate plate titred in identical manner with negative serum may prove necessary in some cases where the antigen has a high affinity for non-specific immunoglobulin. A total lack of colour indicates that the enzyme is wrongly diluted, that the substrate (especially the H_2O_2) was not fresh or that inhibitors such as azide are still present in the buffer. Unexpected colour reactions usually relate to poor blocking or washing (for example residual glutaraldehyde may bind unwanted antibody). Assays for cellular antigens generally give more problems if, for example, the cells have Fc receptors. Some cell types also have residual endogenous peroxidase activity and in these cases alkaline phosphatase or β-galactosidase should be employed (though alkaline phosphatase may also show endogenous activity). Discontinuities in the plate due to thermal gradients may also be observed (Oliver et al., 1981) but these are minimised by the use of incubations at room temperature.

2.6.10. The use of ELISA for screening

Once the appropriate antigen concentration and antibody titre have been determined by the chequerboard assay, screening plates may be set up. These should all be at the chosen antigen density and may be stored at 4 °C, with coating antigen or blocking buffer. Monoclonal antibody supernatants from the tissue culture plates are then added to each well. As discussed in Sections 2.2 and 2.3 it is probably better to allow incubation with the monoclonal antibody to be overnight at 4 °C but otherwise the protocol employed is as in Protocol 2.1 Step (viii) onwards once the hybridoma supernatant has been washed off the plate.

Controls for hybridoma selection are very important. Duplicates are particularly valuable for the confirmation of a weak positive. It is essential not to select antibodies which bind to the plates or the blocking reagents and this means that supernatants should be tested on an identical plate without the antigen. However, the amount of tissue culture supernatant is usually limited and it is possible to select potential positives and rescreen these with the necessary duplicates and controls when more antibody has been released by the cells in culture. Controls without antibody are also necessary for each assay as the background may differ slightly between two assays and it is difficult to select positive samples otherwise.

2.6.11. The dot immunobinding assay

The dot immunobinding assay in which the antigen is attached to nitrocellulose on a series of 'dots' is the natural assay system of choice for screening on a limited budget. It is claimed to be equally sensitive to or more sensitive than ELISA assays. The original method of Hawkes et al. (1982), involved the application of dots of the antigen to nitrocellulose sheets followed by cutting up of the sheets so that square pieces of paper containing the dots were put into the microtitre wells for incubation with the monoclonal antibody. A variation on this involved the inversion of the microtitre plates containing the monoclonal antibody over the sheets with a matrix of dotted antigen with a tight seal for the antibody–antigen incubation (Bennet and Yeoman, 1983). Both these techniques allow the paper-bound antigen to have contact with a large amount of supernatant while the protocol given in Protocol 2.3 does not. However, Protocol 2.3 (derived from Smith et al., 1983) has proved extremely successful and is very simple and it may readily be tested with serum to see whether or not it suits the antibody–antigen system under examination. (See Addendum.)

An interesting variation on the dot assay used by Locker and Motta (1983) involves the covalent binding of the hybridoma supernatant to DBM (diazotized aminobenzyloxymethyl) paper. This is then incubated with solution of radioactive antigen, washed and counted. The attractive features of this assay are the direct nature with no sandwiches, and the covalent attachment of the antibody. However, the requirement for labelling of the antigen limits the general application.

Protocol 2.3

Dot immunobinding chequerboard assay for soluble antigens

(i) Immunise a rat or mouse with antigen (Chapter 5). Boost 4–7 days before bleeding but not killing the animal. Withdraw 0.1–0.2 ml serum. Prepare stock negative serum from an unimmunised mouse of the same strain and age.

(ii) Rule out 6 × 6 squares of 9 mm on a sheet of nitrocellulose paper using a paper template on a light box. Wash the piece of paper in distilled water and dry at room temperature for at least 1 h. Make up doubling dilutions of antigen over the range 1 mg/ml, 0.5 mg/ml, 0.25 mg/ml, 0.125 mg/ml and 0.063 mg/ml. Leave the last column with no antigen.

(iii) Using a Hamilton syringe pipette 1 μl of the highest concentration of antigen as a dot into the centre of each square in the first column. Pipette 1 μl of the second concentration into the centre of each square in the second column and so on until the sixth column has 1 μl in each square at the highest dilution. The dried sheet may be stored over a considerable period of time in the case of most antigens.

(iv) Incubate the paper in 10 mg/ml bovine serum albumin or 1% bovine serum in a small container such as the lid of a 96-well microtitre plate for 15 min to block the reactive sites. Blot the paper dry gently.

(v) Make up dilutions of antiserum at 1/50, 1/100, 1/200, 1/500 and 1/1000. Make up negative serum at 1/50. Pipette 1–2 µl of the lowest dilution (highest concentration) onto each of the antigen dots the first row, 1–2 µl of the next concentration onto the second row and so on. Put 1–2 µl of the negative serum in the sixth row. Incubate for only 3–5 min and then wash the paper five times in PBS.

(vi) Incubate the paper with horseradish peroxidase conjugated anti mouse (or rat) IgG diluted 1 in 100 with PBS containing 0.5 mg/ml BSA. Wash again five times with PBS.

(vii) To develop the colour mix 1 volume of a stock solution of 3 mg/ml 4-chloro-1-naphthol (Sigma) dissolved in methanol and stored in the dark with 5 volumes of PBS and H_2O_2 to 0.01%. Blue colouration should appear on the bound antibody complexes after 5–15 min. Wash the filter with distilled water and store in the dark. The paper should appear like the ELISA assay to have strong colour in the top left-hand corner and no staining in the bottom right-hand one. The titre of the animal serum and the most suitable concentration of antigen to employ during screening can then be evaluated.

2.6.12. Screening with the dot immunobinding assay

It will be evident from the simplicity of the process that it is possible to screen large numbers of antibodies by dot immunobinding in a short period of time and at minimal cost. If sufficient concentrations of antigen are not contained in 1 µl it is possible to make several applications of a dilute solution allowing the paper to dry each time. In order to add more antibody it is possible to use the aluminium template described by Smith et al. (1984) to increase both the volume and time of the incubation or to use an inverted microtitre plate as described by Bennet and Yeoman (1983). However, the *antibody* must *not* be allowed to dry on the paper. It should be noted that Smith et al. (1983) were detecting rat monoclonal antibodies which can be assayed at a later stage when the antibody concentration in the medium is comparatively high since there is less urgency for subcloning (Chapter 3). (See also Addendum.)

2.7. Soluble-phase systems

The soluble-phase system most commonly employed for hybridoma screening is a radioimmunoassay. Radioimmunoassay is a widely employed term and is often used to describe the solid-phase binding assay described in Section 2.6 where radiolabelled rather than enzyme-linked second antibody is employed.

Soluble-phase assays are generally less convenient for screening because of the requirement for large amounts of labelled antigen. However, they may well be the wisest method of choice where the final application of the antibody is to be in a soluble-phase assay. Miller et al. (1983) have shown that antibodies selected on a solid phase assay can yield false positive hybridomas whose antibodies do not react with the antigen in solution. Conversely, antibodies selected in a solution-phase assay do not always react in a solid-phase assay. The phenomenon probably relates to the exposure of different antigen epitopes in binding to the solid phase, although radiolabelling of the antigen may also play some part.

It is suggested (Thomson, 1982) that soluble-phase assays such as radioimmunoassay will become obsolete as the IRMA assays (Fig. 2.3) utilising two monoclonal antibodies of different epitope specificity become more widely used. However, where radioimmunoassays are directed towards small molecules such as steroid hormones, it seems unlikely that they can be superceded in this manner.

In most soluble-phase assays the main technical problem lies in separating free from bound antigen. This is most conveniently performed by the use of a second antibody linked to a solid phase. Second antibodies bound to Sepharose 4B are commercially available (Pharmacia). The monoclonal antibody is reacted directly with a radioactive antigen and the complex is then separated from unreacted antigen using the Sepharose-bound antibody and then counted.

2.8. Cellular assays

Antibodies associated with cell-surface antigens may be selected by a solid-phase assay as described in Section 2.6. However, sometimes monoclonal antibodies are required not only to bind to cells but also to perform specific functions. For example, blood grouping antibodies are usually selected by haemagglutination because this is the technique in which they are likely to be finally employed. Similarly antibodies required for cytotoxicity purposes can be screened by direct determination of this property. These screening systems are generally less sensitive and a good general protocol is to isolate the antibodies of interest in a primary solid-phase screen and test this much smaller number in a subsequent cellular assay. It should, however, be noted that the glutaraldehyde fixation routinely employed in solid-phase assays of cells may destroy some epitopes on the antigen. A simple assay for cells not bound to a solid phase can be performed in a microtitre plate which has been first blocked with 200 μl of 10 mg/ml bovine serum albumin. 100 μl of the monoclonal antibody and 50 μl of cells at a concentration of 10^5 to 10^6 cells/ml are then mixed and incubated in the wells. After 2–3 h at room temperature the plate is centrifuged for 5 min at 400 g (in special plate holders or taped to the sample holder of a bench centrifuge). The supernatant is removed with a *single* flick of the plate (it is all too easy to dislodge cells from the pellet) and the cells are washed in PBS containing 0.5 mg/ml BSA. The labelled or enzyme-linked second antibody is then added for the second incubation and the plate is again washed. The radioactivity in the wells is then determined or assayed for enzyme activity according to the procedures in Protocol 2.2. The advantage of this procedure is that the properties of the cells have not been altered by fixation to a solid surface. The disadvantages are that the washing procedures may result in loss of cells and that the cells cannot be stored.

Direct haemagglutination assays are generally performed by adding 50 µl monoclonal antibody to 25 µl of 1% v/v suspensions of red blood cells suspended in PBS containing 10 mg/ml BSA and incubating at room temperature for 1–2 h. For indirect haemagglutination the cells are washed and resuspended in 50 µl of anti-mouse IgG and incubated for a further hour (Fraser et al., 1982). The method is used largely for erythrocyte membrane antigens but can be used for screening any soluble protein attached to sheep red blood cells by Protocol 7.2.

Rosetting assays have also been employed in hybridoma analysis (Mosmann et al., 1980; Koo and Goldberg, 1978) but are generally regarded as too cumbersome for screening.

Cytotoxicity assays are usually performed in Terasaki microculture plates. Typically 2 µl of monoclonal antibody are mixed with 1 µl of target cells and 4 µl of rabbit or guinea pig complement and incubated at room temperature for an hour. The cells are then stained with 10 µl of 0.1% trypan blue in saline and inspected for viability (Hammerling et al., 1981).

Many of the early monoclonal antibody experiments were to antibodies against sheep red blood cells. In these situations it was possible to overlay clones growing in agar with the antigen and complement and select clones from the visible plaques (Kohler and Milstein, 1978).

2.9. Biological assays

Biological assays in hybridoma screening are very unusual and generally avoided because they take too long and are cumbersome to carry out in large numbers. However, the first highly successful antibody to interferon was made in this way (Secher and Burke, 1980). Other more frequently employed biochemical assays are used when an antibody which is directed to the active site of an enzyme is screened for its effect on enzyme activity. Antibodies to hormone receptors can also be screened for their ability to block the binding of the hormone to the receptor. The antibody selected in this way may of course be exerting its biological effect by a more long range mechanism than physical blocking of the active site.

2.10. Immunocytochemical assays

This type of assay is obviously not convenient for the screening of a large number of samples. However, as with the cellular assays, if the final use of the monoclonal antibody is to be in such an assay then it is advisable to perform a second screen of hybridoma supernatants which are positive in a solid-phase-binding assay at an early stage. The fixatives used in particular for tissue sections can have dramatic effects on the availability of various determinants so that no reaction or a reaction of quite different specificity may be found in the immunocytochemical assay (Milstein et al., 1983). Frozen tissue sections can also show a very different reaction from fixed ones and it is useful to assay with tissue sections prepared in as many different ways as possible.

Immunohistochemical assays have the obvious advantage of giving direct evidence relating not only to the presence of the antigen but also its cellular distribution.

Antibodies may be screened either by fluorescent or by enzyme-linked second antibodies. While a variety of enzymes have been used, horseradish peroxidase is by far the preferred linked enzyme because of the ease with which the reaction product may be demonstrated by microscopy (reviewed by Farr and Nakane, 1981). However, biotin-conjugated second antibodies (Bayer and Wilcheck, 1980) which are then detected by avidin-conjugated dye or fluorochrome are also an exceptionally good system. Biotinylation causes minimal damage to the antibody and the use of the carcinogenic peroxidase substrates is avoided.

Cells rather than fixed tissue sections may be used in the procedure described in Section 2.8 using a microtitre plate and centrifuging the cells between washes. This is particularly suitable for screening for cell-surface antigens. A fluorescent second antibody is used in place of the enzyme labelled one and 0.1% sodium azide is incorporated into the buffer to reduce antigen capping. The hazards involved in losing cells are less serious in this procedure as a quantitative estimate is not required. Once the cells have been reacted with the second antibody and washed, they are transferred to multisample slides and fixed in cold alcohol, methanol or acetone for 5 min and dried.

Target cells may also be fixed on slides before incubation with the antibody. This method allows antibodies to intracellular components to be detected. The cells are grown overnight on multiwell slides or fixed by incubation for 30 min on multiwell slides which have been pretreated with 50 µg/ml poly-L-lysine. The excess binding capacity of the polylysine is then blocked with a drop of 10 mg/ml bovine serum albumin. The slides are fixed in methanol, ethanol or alcohol for 5 min and can be washed and stored.

Incubation with the hybridoma supernatant is carried out in a humidified box for up to 1 h and the antibody is then removed and the slide washed in phosphate-buffered saline three times. A drop of fluorescent labelled or enzyme-linked second antibody is then added and the slides are again incubated in a humidified atmosphere for 30 min. After washing, the slides are then viewed in a fluorescent microscope or reacted with the substrate according to whether a fluorescent or enzyme-labelled second antibody has been used. The usual substrate for peroxidase assays is 0.05% 3,3'-diaminobenzidine in PBS containing 0.03% H_2O_2 which is a carcinogen and must be handled with care. The slides are incubated in a solution of this for 30 min, washed and inspected under the microscope.

CHAPTER 3

Selection of animals and cell lines

3.1. Choice of animal

There are three systems currently utilised for monoclonal antibody production. These are mouse, rat and human. It is not possible to make hybridomas from rabbits as suitable myeloma cell lines are not readily generated in these animals. Human hybridomas are at an early stage of development and their use is generally only contemplated in the specialised cases described below (Section 3.6).

However both mouse and rat systems are widely used and the choice between the two is a fairly open one. An elementary consideration which is self evident relates to the nature of the antigen. As in conventional antibody production, the more foreign the antigen the better the response is likely to be. The rat is not generally employed for the production of antibodies to a rat protein except in specialised cases where autoimmune phenomena are being investigated, and a mouse is not used for murine antigens. Even in these cases, however, the variation between strains within a species can allow exceptions to this general rule to be employed. With an antigen of neither rat nor mouse origin, the response of the two species can still vary greatly in vigour and a few preliminary experiments on both may indicate that one or other is an obvious choice for satisfactory hybridoma production. Cross-species fusions using mouse myloma cells and spleen cells from a rat immunised with murine antigens have also been performed (Cotton and Milstein, 1973; Galfre et al., 1977; Springer et al., 1978; Ledbetter and Herzenberg, 1979).

The mouse system was historically the first to be developed as a method for the production of monoclonal antibodies of predefined specificity (Kohler and Milstein, 1975) and the majority of hybridomas described to date are of mouse origin. However, the rat system has been reported to have definite advantages. The reversion of the parent lines to non-secreting forms is lower than in the mouse cell lines available (under 10^{-4}/cell/generation against 10^{-3}/cell/generation) and this is obviously a valuable characteristic if it is retained in the fusion progeny. An additional though possibly related advantage in the rat system is that 90% of the growing fusion hybrids express spleen immunoglobulins where the mouse system shows only 60% (Clark et al., 1983). Rats are also larger and can yield approximately 10 times more ascitic fluid in the production stages (Galfre et al., 1979). Additional advantages of the rat system may lie in the production of a high frequency of antibodies able to fix human complement. This property may be significant if therapeutic applications are envisaged. One reported minor disadvantage of the rat system relates to the comparatively low affinity of most rat immunoglobulins for protein A which is therefore not so frequently a suitable agent for subsequent purification (Ledbetter and Herzenberg, 1979). However, affinity for protein A seems to be a highly individual property of each monoclonal antibody (Chapter 9) and at least some rat IgG molecules can be purified on Protein A (Rousseaux et al., 1981) (Section 9.7.2).

3.2. Choice of cell lines

There are several desirable characteristics in a good myeloma line as fusion partner some of which occasionally conflict. The major ones are discussed below. The suppliers are either established commercial laboratories such as Flow or Gibco or the ATCC (American Type Culture Collection) (Appendix 2).

3.2.1. Myeloma antibody synthesis

It is clearly preferable in a fusion experiment to use a myeloma partner which does not itself make antibody. If this is not the case then hybridomas can result which produce antibodies with a variety of mixtures of chains giving lower overall affinity and possibly non-standard affinity and specificity if there are differential alterations in the synthesis of the chains (Fig. 3.1.a). If the myeloma makes only a light chain then the amount of irrelevant antibody is limited and at least 25 % of the immunoglobulin produced will be of the desired specifici-

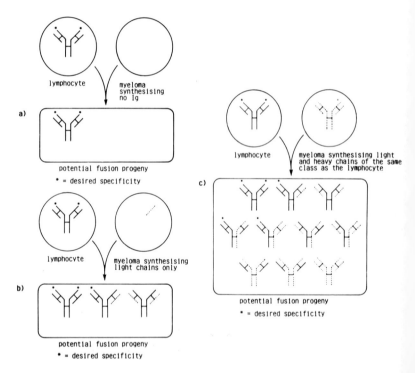

Fig. 3.1. The advantage of using a non-secreting myeloma parent cell line. (a) The progeny secrete antibodies of the desired specificity. (b) The output of the progeny cell lines is diluted by antibodies carrying the irrelevant myeloma kappa chain. (c) If the parent myeloma cell line secretes antibodies of the same class as the fusion partner then there is considerable dilution of secreted antibody with hybrid molecules of irrelevant specificity. Subclones which have lost the ability to secrete some of these antibodies may be isolated but this adds greatly to the experimental workload.

ty (Fig. 3.1.b). However, if both parent myeloma and lymphocyte synthesise heavy chains of the same class then the dilution of specific antibody made by the hybridoma is considerable. With hybridomas which secrete low amounts of antibody, this is particularly relevant as much of the energy of the cell is directed into the production of unusable material (Fig. 3.1.c). In the mouse system it has been shown that hybrid molecules can be formed between different IgG subclasses although they do not form between the heavy chains of IgG and IgM (Kohler et al., 1978). Various types of hybrid molecules have also been reported in early cross-species fusions (Schwaber and Cohen, 1974). At the moment several mouse myeloma lines, one rat line (or more, see Section 3.4) and no human lines free of antibody secretion are available.

3.2.2. Hybridoma antibody secretion

Despite the fact that it should not make antibody itself, the myeloma cell line employed for fusion should lead to clones secreting large amounts of antibody. Clearly a parent fusion line which has any defects in its ability to make or secrete all immunoglobulins rather than its own particular (and unwanted) one would be an unsuitable fusion partner. In theory, a plasmocytoma cell line derived from a tumour which has the ability to secrete large amounts of antibody should therefore be superior to a lymphoblastoid cell line. Much has been written about this aspect of the myeloma lines available for fusion but few good statistical studies have been performed and it is worth noting the work of Cote et al. (1983) who showed that using two human and one mouse fusion partners a range of hybridomas varying 100-fold in their secretion ability could be generated from each line and none of the cell lines could be shown to be superior in this particular respect. Figures are usually given in µg immunoglobulin secreted by 10^6 cells in 24 h and published papers do not always express data in these units so comparisons are difficult. Figures can vary widely from below 1 µg to over 100 µg.

3.2.3. Hybridisation frequency

The cell line employed in fusion should ideally lead to a high frequency of clones of fused cells. This parameter varies quite widely among research groups and, within groups, among particular experiments. No detailed comparisons of all available cell lines against a single type of antigen are available and much of the evidence is anecdotal. Even with two halves of the same spleen from an immunised animal it is difficult to obtain a valid comparison since the two fusions must necessarily involve either two operators or a time delay between the two experiments. However, in general mouse myelomas should yield hybridisation frequencies in the broad range of 1–100 clones per 10^7 lymphocytes and human hybridisation frequencies are about an order of magnitude lower. Frequency of fusion will also depend on the ratio of the two types of fused cells and the nature and purity of the lymphocytes used to partner the myeloma in the fusion.

3.2.4. Reversion frequency

The importance of reversion frequency is mentioned above in Section 3.1 in relation to the rat system. With established hybridomas reversion is usually a rare phenomenon and it is readily overcome by routine subcloning so the advantage is small. It is in the selection from the primary fusion of suitable clones for subcloning that the advantage of the rat system is a very major one. In general, cells which lose the power to secrete antibody, will overgrow any neighbours still secreting it so that in the early stages of selection, good clones are frequently swamped and lost. The lower reversion frequency makes this very much less likely and consequently useful clones are more readily established (Clark et al., 1983). This parameter is not readily measured in parent myelomas which are non-secretors. However, with those which do secrete antibody it is a useful guide as to the potential behaviour of the progeny (Section 3.1). While no systematic studies have been published, the reversion rate of the actual fused cells is more relevant and the most suitable cell line is one in which a high proportion of the wells which are positive at the first screening remain positive thereafter. This could relate to the speed of chromosome loss in hybrids rather than the properties of the parent line.

3.3. Selective drug markers

3.3.1. HAT medium

It is vital that the parent cell line can be selected against in tissue culture so that non-fused cells may be eliminated from the fusion mixture. The commonest method for carrying out this procedure is to use a parent myeloma which has been selected for its sensitivity to

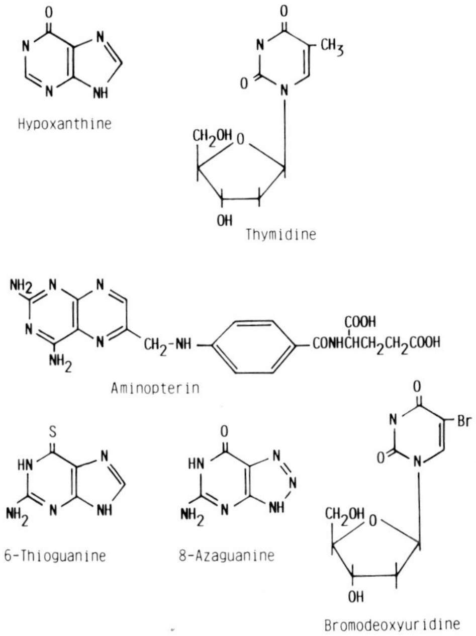

Fig. 3.2. The structure of some of the common chemicals involved in the selection and use of HAT-sensitive cells.

Hypoxanthine, Aminopterin (or Amethopterin) and Thymidine (HAT) medium (Fig. 3.2). Figure 3.3 shows the manner in which the selection procedure works. Aminopterin (and also Amethopterin) block the main biosynthetic pathways for purine and pyrimidine synthesis in animal cells principally by inhibition of the enzyme dihydrofolate reductase. There are, however, salvage pathways by which exogenous nucleosides may be utilised instead. The pyrimidine pathway involves the enzyme thymidine kinase (TK) and utilises exogenous thymidine. The purine pathways utilises the enzyme hypoxanthine (guanine) phosphoribosyl transferase [H(G)PRT] with exogenous hypoxanthine. Cell lines can be made deficient in either one of these enzymes by growth and selection in either bromodeoxyuridine (which selects TK negative cells) or azaguanine or thioguanine (which select HGPRT negative cells). In normal cells these inhibitors are converted to the appropriate nucleotides which are cytotoxic and consequently only mutants deficient in the appropriate enzymes survive. Nearly all the rodent cell lines currently in use have been selected in azaguanine and are consequently HPRT negative. Commercial

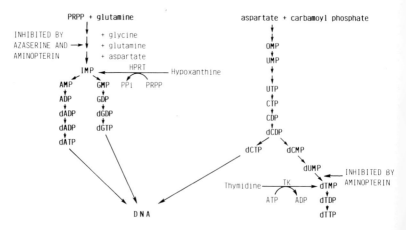

Fig. 3.3. The main pathways of purine and pyrimidine biosynthesis and major sites of aminopterin and azaserin blockage. Azaserine may also inhibit pyrimidine biosynthesis but at comparatively higher concentrations.

constraints are such that, particularly with the human system, it is sometimes expedient to select an HPRT or TK negative cell line in the laboratory rather than acquire one from other sources.

3.3.2. Selection for azaguanine, thioguanine and bromodeoxyuridine resistant mutants

In general it is easier to select for HPRT negative cells rather than for TK negative ones. In most mammals, the chromosomal locus is on the X chromosome and whatever the sex of the original tumour donor, only one X chromosome is generally transcriptionally active in established cell lines. Consequently only one mutation is required in theory for an HPRT negative mutant to be generated. 6-Thioguanine is probably better than 8-azaguanine for the selection of HPRT negative mutants (Evans and Vijayalaxmi, 1981). The latter is reported to be incorporated into RNA as well as DNA which effectively protects cells against its mutagenic effect (Nelson et al., 1975). More importantly, nearly all mutants selected in thioguanine are HPRT negative whereas selection in azaguanine can lead to the production of cell lines with normal levels of the enzyme (Littlefield, 1963; Cox and Masson, 1978). Cells are selected in gradually increasing concentrations starting at around 1 µg/ml (it is a good idea to vary this within a small range as different cell types may show different sensitivity) and leading up to levels from 30 to 100 µg/ml after 6–8 weeks. The cells may be mutagenised first with irradiation or treatment with ethyl methanesulphonate but this is not necessary. If there is extensive cell death, the surviving cells can be purified on Ficoll. The resistant cells are cloned several times in soft agar or by limiting dilution and clones are chosen for high growth rate and low reversion frequency to growth in HAT medium. TK negative cell lines are selected in a similar way with bromodeoxyuridine as the selective agent.

3.3.3. Selection for ouabain-resistant mutants

Ouabain resistance is a convenient additional property, particularly where human cell lines are employed. Rodent cell lines grow in levels of ouabain up to 10^{-3} M where human ones generally die at levels of 10^{-7} M so that in human–rodent fusions ouabain can be used as a selective agent against the unfused human cells. To prepare a human ouabain-resistant mutant it is usual but not essential to mutagenise the cells with irradiation (100–200 R) or with mutagens such as ethyl methanesulphonate (100 µg/ml). The cells are then selected with ouabain levels increasing from 10^{-7} M gradually over a period of several weeks. This procedure has been particularly useful for fusion of EB transformed cell lines (Kozbor et al., 1982).

3.3.4. Other methods of selection

Other methods of selection of cells involve the use of different selective medium, the use of irreversible inhibitors, or the Fluorescence Activated Cell Sorter (FACS). Selective medium containing hypoxanthine and azaserine can be used for azaguanine or thioguanine resistant mutants. Azaserine blocks the pathways of purine biosynthesis but not pyrimidine biosynthesis (Fig. 3.3) and consequently thymidine need not be included in the medium. Thymidine inhibits DNA synthesis at millimolar concentrations in most mammalian cells and some cell types are susceptible at lower concentrations. Hypoxanthine and azaserine containing selective medium is therefore often involved. This is especially true in human fusions and azaserine is frequently employed in both human B cell fusions (Edwards et al., 1982) and T cell fusions (Foung et al., 1982).

Irreversible inhibitors have not yet been shown to be a completely suitable method of establishing hybridomas. However, it is a potentially valuable system for fusing any two cell types which have not been previously selected for drug resistance. In essence the procedure involves the use of an irreversible poison of a different type on both of the two cells to be fused. They can then only survive by fusion.

It is thought that this system may be of value for the production of T cell hybridomas because of their extreme sensitivity to thymidine (Kobayashi et al., 1982).

Selection by the FACS is discussed in more detail in Chapters 6 and 7.

3.4. The mouse system

Table 3.1 lists the mouse cell lines currently available as fusion partners.

TABLE 3.1
Suitable mouse cell lines for fusion

Cell line	Immunoglobulin expression	Derived from	Reference
P3-X63/Ag 8	gamma, kappa	MOPC-21	1
NSI/1.Ag 4.1	kappa (non-secreted)	MOPC-21	2
X63/Ag 8.653	none	X63-Ag8	3
Sp2/O	none	Hybridoma Sp2	4
NSO/U	none	HSI/1.Ag4.1	3
FO	none	Clone of Sp2/O	5
MPC11-X45-6TG1.7	gamma$_{2b}$, kappa	Balb/c	6
S194/5XXO Bul	none	Balb/c	7

References
1 Kohler, G., and Milstein, C. (1975) Nature 256, 495.
2 Kohler, G., Howe, S.C., and Milstein, C. (1976) Eur. J. Immunol. 6, 292.
3 Kearney, J.F., Radbruch, A., Liesegang, B., and Rajewsky, K. (1979) J. Immunol. 123, 1548.
4 Shulman, M., Wilde, C.D., and Kohler, G. (1978) Nature 276, 269.
5 Fazekas de St. Groth, S., and Scheidegger, D. (1980) J. Immunol. Meth. 35, 1.
6 Margulies, D.H., Kuehl, W.M., and Scharff, M.D. (1976) Cell 8, 405.
7 Trowbridge, I. (1978) J. Exp. Med. 148, 313.

All the cell lines originated in Balb/c mice. It can be seen that suitable cell lines are either produced by the selection of subclones from a normal parent line or from the selection of a hybridoma cell line itself. Suppliers of the first four cell lines in Table 3.1 are Flow Laboratories Ltd., Irvine, Ayrshire, Scotland, and other branches or the laboratory which first produced the line itself. Now that the commercial potential of hybridomas is becoming clearer, it is common for a laboratory to ask the recipient to sign a form of words indicating that the profits from any commercially valuable hybridoma produced by use of the cell lines will be suitably apportioned.

The most obvious choice of mouse strain for immunisation is Balb/c since this is compatible with all the available parent myeloma cell lines and consequently the hybridomas produced can be grown subsequently in ascitic fluid. However there is considerable variation in the immune response of different inbred mouse strains to different antigens and if a poor response is shown by a Balb/c strain then other strains should be assessed for a more vigorous one. If SJL mouse spleen cells are used for the fusion because SJL mice respond well, then the resulting hybridoma should be propagated in ascitic fluid in vivo in an F1 hybrid of Balb/c and SJL. Propagation in ascitic fluid

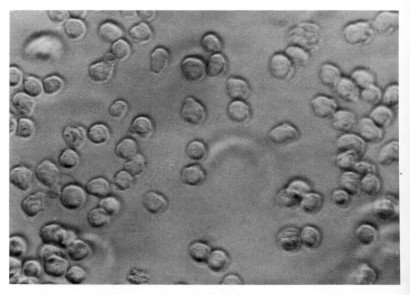

Fig. 3.4. Typical mouse myeloma X63/Ag. 8 653 cells in culture (magnification × 1000).

is not an essential part of hybridoma production however and many laboratories prefer to culture on large scale in vitro (Chapter 9). An alternative to immunising a totally incompatible strain is to immunise the F1 hybrid itself and use their spleen cells in the fusion. Poor antigens very often evoke a more vigorous response in SJL or NZB mice and their Balb/c F1 hybrids and it is worth spending time testing a few mouse strains for their suitability before proceeding with fusions. Some of the main characteristics of the most frequently used mouse strains are given in Festing (1979). Mice should be obtained from a reputable supplier who employs regular routine tests of genetic quality control as one white mouse looks very like another to the average laboratory worker. A list of recommended suppliers can be obtained from the Medical Research Council Laboratory Animals Centre, Woodmansterne Road, Carshalton, Surrey SM5 4EF. This facility is shortly to be curtailed and in the near future enquiries will be better made to Mr. Alan Smith, Laboratory Animals Breeders Association, Charles River, U.K. Ltd., Manston Research Centre, Manston Road, Margate, Kent. In the U.K. it is necessary to hold Home Office Licences (Appendix 1).

3.5. The rat system

Some of the advantages of the rat system have already been discussed is Section 3.1. The rat system was originally developed by Bazin (Bazin et al., 1972, 1973; see Bazin, 1982 for background). Rat myelomas are comparatively rare and two strains of rat were developed in Louvain by Bazin's group in the 1970s. Lou/C rats have a high incidence of ileocaecal tumours and Lou-M strains a low one. The tumours show the characteristics of plasmocytomas. One of these myeloma cell lines which Bazin refers to as the S210 was developed in the U.K. as the R210 line and clones which were azaguanine-resistant and which were good fusion partners were isolated. There are two related cell lines of this type available in the U.K., both based on the R210.RCY3 cell line from Lou/C rats. The Y3-Ag 1.2.3 cell line

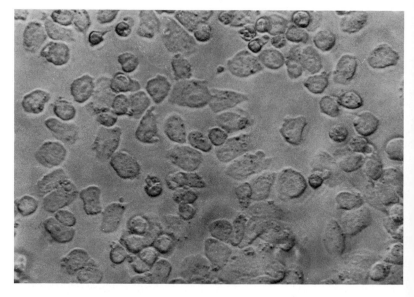

Fig. 3.5. Typical rat myeloma Y3 Ag.1.2.3 cells in culture (magnification × 1000).

(Galfre et al., 1979) secretes a kappa chain and the YB2/3 Ag20 which is a myeloma line derived from a fusion between the original Y3 line and the spleen cells from an AO rat immunised with human complement, secretes and makes no immunoglobulin (Lachman et al., (1980). They can be obtained from the Medical Research Council Laboratory of Molecular Biology, Hills Road, Cambridge CB2 2QH if the appropriate consent forms are signed. However, in Belgium Bazin (1983) has also developed an azaguanine-resistant non-secreting line IR983F. The Belgian myeloma lines are no longer histocompatible with the U.K. lines despite their common origin (Bazin, personal communication).

It is obviously preferable (though not essential) that the rat to be immunised should be of the Lou strain as well and these can be obtained in Belgium from H. Bazin, Experimental Immunology Unit, Bte UCl 3056, Clos Chapelle Aux Champs 30, 1200 Brussels, Belgium and in the U.K. from OLAC (1976) Ltd., Shaw's Farm, Blackthorn,

Bicester OX6 OTP. Again, the U.K. rats are compatible with the UK Y3 cell line and the Belgian rats with the original parent cell lines but rats from the two countries cannot be used for the propagation of the foreign cell lines. In the U.K. the lack of availability of Lou rats in recent years has led to many people immunising the DA strain which is readily available. Hybridomas should then be propagated in the F1 hybrids of Lou and DA and this has the advantage that the search for the Lou rat can be postponed until the necessity is established. Hybrids can be ultimately propagated in the DA strain alone, especially with preliminary irradiation, if Lou rats remain unavailable. Alternatively, all attempts to propagate in ascites may be abandoned and the hybridoma may be grown in bulk cell culture (Chapter 9).

3.6. The human system

3.6.1. Introduction

It must be emphasised that human hybridomas are very much harder to make than rodent ones and it is probably not wise to attempt to make them unless the final application of the monoclonal antibody precludes the use of mouse or rat (Edwards and O'Hare, 1984). There is no non-secreting human myeloma or lymphoblastoid cell line available and this leads to mixed and diluted antibody production (Section 3.2.1, Fig. 3.3). While hybrids of the appropriate specificity are sometimes obtained after the initial fusion experiment, subcloning presents many technical difficulties. The initial results can therefore lead to much unjustified optimism since if the rodent system can be taken as a suitable model, the hybridoma will eventually stop secreting unless it is subcloned. Consequently, if the human immune response at a specific point in time is to be amplified for further limited investigation, the human system can be utilised, but if the establishment of a permanent cell line is the main goal then this is exceptionally hard to achieve.

3.6.2. Immunisation

Immunisation is dealt with in greater detail in Chapter 4. In general humans are not specifically immunised for monoclonal antibody production unless routine vaccines such as tetanus are employed. Human hybridomas are of interest more for the study of the human response to autoimmune or malignant disease and the amplification and dissection of this response. However, vaccination with routine pathogens or their toxins gives a ready source of suitable human lymphocytes. The effective 'background' is also reduced by the use of the human system where a self response is investigated since the fact that the human material is foreign to a mouse may mask the more relevant antigenic response. Thus a patient's response to their own tumour is probably more relevant than a murine response to injected human tumour cells where the fusion may be dominated by antigens related to histocompatibility rather than malignancy. While it is often impractical to seek human volunteers for immunisation with some agents, the possibility of in vitro immunisation with lymphoid tissue has often been considered. Human tonsils and spleens are often readily available for this type of experiment, though the former encompass some risk of mycoplasma infection in the cell cultures. In vitro immunisation has been the subject of intensive investigation and there is no doubt that incubation with the antigen can lead to an increased response (reviewed in Reading, 1982, see Chapter 4). However, there are no well documented cases of an in vitro response to a completely foreign antigen (in humans) and it seems likely that the cells will only respond to antigen to which the whole individual has previously presented an immune response.

3.6.3. Cell lines

The available cell lines for human monoclonal antibody production are well reviewed by Kozbor and Roder (1983). Early fusion experiments were often carried out with the mouse cell lines described in Section 3.3 as good human cell lines were not available. These interspecies hybrids tend to preferentially lose human chromosomes though human chromosome 14 (which carries the heavy chain locus) and 22 (which carries the lambda locus) are frequently retained (Croce et al., 1980). The likely instability of mouse–human hybrid means that they are not favoured as a method of making human monoclonal antibodies. In addition, loss of secretion even in clones retaining the appropriate chromosomes has been observed (Raison et al., 1982). Nevertheless Cote et al. (1983) have shown that if early and repeated subcloning is carried out, the mouse–human system yields hybridomas with stability comparable to human–human fusions and it may be that the early attempts were not strenuous enough. The use of the mouse system means that it is possible to employ non-secreting cell lines which is not yet possible with human hybridomas and problems relating to Epstein Barr virus (see Section 3.6.4) are also minimised. The use of a mouse plasmocytoma partner is therefore well worth consideration.

There are four main human cell lines available (see also Addendum) for use in human–human fusions and these are detailed below (see Edwards and O'Hare, 1984, for more detail and Abrams et al., 1983, and Cote et al., 1983, for comparisons). It is advisable to check the karyotypes of all human cell lines received from elsewhere (Section 10.5).

SKO-007 (U-266AR1)

This cell line was the first to be used for human monoclonal antibody production (Olsson and Kaplan, 1980). It is azaguanine-resistant and secretes the epsilon heavy chain and lambda light chain. It is negative for Epstein Barr Nuclear Antigen (EBNA) and can be obtained from Becton Dickinson, Sunnyvale, California. The line showed some problems with mycoplasma infection in the early 1980s but this has now been successfully removed. SK-007 is of plasmocytoma origin and might therefore be expected to secrete more substantial amounts of antibody than some of the other cell lines available. However, if a large number of hybridomas are studied (Cote et al., 1983) the amount of immunoglobulin secreted can vary 100-fold among clones with this and other cell lines as fusion partners. Reported fusion frequencies range up to 40 clones/10^7 lymphocytes but the median is very much at the lower end of the range.

GM1500-6TG-2

GM1500 is a thioguanine-resistant lymphoblastoid cell line secreting a gamma-2b heavy chain and kappa light chain. It carries the Epstein Barr Nuclear Antigen. Reported fusion frequencies range up to 25×10^{-7}. This line can be obtained from The Wistar Institute, Philadelphia. A subline of this, the GM4672, has been successfully used to produce hybridomas from patients with various autoimmune conditions (Shoenfeld et al., 1982, 1983) and was obtained from the Cell Repository, Institute of Medical Research, Camden, New Jersey (it is reported to be EBNA negative).

A useful ouabain resistant line derived from GM1500 is the KR-4 line (Kozbor et al., 1982). This line can be fused with human lymphocytes which bear no selective markers since only the progeny which have the ouabain resistance of one parent and the thioguanine resistance of the other will survive in selected medium. The line is reported to give exceptionally high hybridisation frequencies (up to 112×10^{-7}) when fused with EBV transformed cell lines and is a potential method for stabilising and increasing the secretion rate of such lines. It is reported to be available from Dr. D. Kozbor, Department of Microbiology and Immunology, Queen's University, Kingston, Ontario.

LICR-LON-HMy2

This is an azaguanine-resistant lymphoblastoid cell line derived from the ARH77 leukemia line (Edwards et al., 1982). It is Epstein Barr Nuclear Antigen positive and secretes gamma one heavy chains and kappa light chains. Initially, fusion frequencies around 1×10^7 were reported but in their extensive studies Cote et al. (1983) and Abrams et al. (1983) show considerably higher mean figures and find this cell line superior to SK-007 in this respect. The cell line is a robust one with a doubling time of 20 h. DMEM is recommended for tissue culture. The cloning efficiency is 25 %. It is available from The Ludwig Institute of Cancer Research, London Branch.

UC729-6

This is a thioguanine-resistant cell line developed by Royston (Glassy et al., 1983a,b) (University of San Diego, Cancer Centre, La Jolla, California 92093) from the human WIL2 lymphoblastoid cell line and is reported to be one of the better lines available for human fusions. It is an IgM kappa secretor. It is readily available if the appropriate consent forms are signed. A small charge (215 dollars) must be paid for processing costs.

An additional human cell line RH-L4 is reported by Olsson et al. (1983). It produces but does not secrete gamma heavy chains and kappa light chains and is EBNA negative. The availability is not clear. It is difficult to recommend any one of these cell lines as a superior fusion partner to any other as the number of stable hybridomas produced from any of them is small.

3.6.4. The Epstein Barr virus transformation system

The EB system is a very attractive method for the production of human hybridomas and is covered in detail in Chapter 7. The virus transforms normal B lymphocytes from blood or tissue samples thus immortalising them and their capacity for antibody production. In a mixed population of transformed cells, antibody secretion reaches a peak after a few weeks and then tails off either due to overgrowth by cells which have lost the capacity to make antibody or some other less well defined loss of ability to secrete. However, if the transformed cells are cloned at an early stage then it is possible antibody secretion be maintained indefinitely. The technique has the obvious advantage in that all B cells with EB receptors are transformed (this is estimated to be one third of the B cell population). Several successful transformations of this type have been reported with the cell lines continuing to make antibody for periods of well over a year (Kozbor and Roder, 1981; Steinitz and Tamir, 1982; Crawford et al., 1983). It is sometimes suggested that these cell lines are inherently unstable and will eventually cease to make antibody but many have been in culture for as long as some hybridomas made by conventional methodology and they appear to have comparable stability particularly if they are of the IgG class. The KR-4 line has been used to increase both stability and secretion rate of such cell lines (Kozbor et al., 1982).

Epstein Barr virus is a herpes type virus known to be involved in the development of Burkitt's lymphoma in parts of Africa and nasopharyngeal carcinoma in Southern China. However, the majority of the population of both developed and underdeveloped countries experience the virus as a subclinical infection of infectious mononucleosis and thereafter have an immune response to the virus. The U.K. Medical Research Council have designated it as a category C pathogen requiring only routine laboratory microbiological practice and consequently it can be used in most laboratories and it is not considered necessary to have samples tested in blood transfusion laboratories. It seems likely that there will be few objections to the clinical use of the antibodies made from fusions involving such cell lines as immunomodulators such as interferon produced from lymphoblastoid cells of this type and antibodies generated with the LICR-HMy-2 line are employed clinically at the present time. However, suitable purification procedures before in vivo application have been agreed (Crawford et al., 1983b). The EB system is therefore one of the best available at the present time for human hybridoma production. No cell line as such is required but the supernatant from the B 95-8 marmoset line which secretes the virus (Miller and Lipman, 1973) is readily obtained from most virology laboratories. A mycoplasma free line is obviously desirable and many B95-8 strains are positive for this. It should be noted that the DNA stains normally used in testing (Chapter 5) are unsuitable for a cell line secreting a virus and a biological assay to test mycoplasma should be employed (Section 5.4.3).

3.7. T cell lines

T cell hybridomas are in their infancy in both murine and human systems. There are no established T cell rat systems.

3.7.1. Mouse T cell fusion partners: The BW-5147 line

The BW-5147 cell line was derived from the AKR thymoma line and made thioguanine and ouabain resistant HPRT negative by Dr. Robert Hyman of La Jolla. It expresses surface antigens Thy 1.1 and H-2k. Hybrids formed between murine splenic T cells and this line can exhibit suppressor function, or helper function and can be shown to have specificity for individual antigens. Cytolytic functions have been harder to establish but have also been reported (see Hammerling et al., 1981 and Fathman and Fitch, 1982, for extensive symposia). This line has been used in the great majority of murine T cell hybridomas produced to date. Other murine partners are discussed in a review by Beezley and Ruddle (1982).

3.7.2. Human T cell hybridomas: The CEM cell line

The CEM cell line is a human T cell leukemia line commercially available (Flow Laboratories). Various laboratories have isolated azaguanine or thioguanine resistant mutants of this and used them in conventional fusion with human lymphocytes (Foung et al., 1982; Irigoyen et al., 1981; Okada et al., 1982). The parent CEM line has also been used in fusions, in the presence of irreversible inhibitors (Kobayashi et al., 1982). Other T cell lines such as Molt-4 are commercially available.

CHAPTER 4

Immunisation

4.1. Introduction

In theory, the immune system of any animal is potentially totipotent. With a broad enough screening system it should be possible to detect antibodies to any antigen which has the potential to elicit a response. Thus spleen cells from non-immunised animals can and have been used for the production of weak hybridomas, and conversely, monoclonal antibodies to materials not in the immunising material can be produced unexpectedly. The commonest of these are monoclonal antibodies to the assay plates themselves or other components of the assay mixture such as the bovine serum albumin used to block the assay plates. The analogy is with the screening of a recombinant genomic DNA library of a particular species for a known gene. However, it is in general unrealistic to hope to select a particular lymphocyte clone from 10^8 to 10^9 others and there is no direct parallel with the genetic selection principles where preliminary enrichment for the chosen gene is by totally different methodology. There is no doubt that the bulk of hybridomas produced to date have arisen from spleens of animals with a high titre of serum antibody, and it is foolish to hope that an antibody of the desired specificity will be obtained from an animal with no immunisation. If the antigen is an agent which infects the animal such as a bacterium or parasite then immunisation may be performed by infection.

It is of interest to note the immense variation in immunisation schedules in published review articles and original papers and consequently the information detailed here must only be regarded as a general guideline. Few systematic studies have been performed as yet and some basic concepts should be stated before any recommendations are made. The very large number of frequently conflicting considerations in these concepts explains to some extent the lack of any coherent and reliable schedule for the production of antibodies to antigens of any specific physical type.

4.1.1. The use of previously established immunisation schedules

No two antigens can be presumed to elicit the same quantitative immune response, however similar they be in physicochemical terms. Published information usually relates to hybridomas already generated. By following the same schedule, with the same antigen, using the same strain of animal and source of lymphocytes, the same myeloma line and the same fusion protocol utilising chemicals from the same supplier, one is likely to generate a very similar panel of hybridomas as in the published work if all such details are indeed supplied. In some cases it is necessary to duplicate experiments to re-establish a lost clone which has ceased to secrete. However, many research groups do not want to duplicate the results of other groups as they are seeking different epitopes or affinities.

In the case of an antigen which may be expected to give the same degree of immune response because of apparently similar physicochemical properties (for example a small molecular weight soluble protein), a totally different response may be elicited because of other factors, for example the variability of carbohydrate residues on glycoproteins or the degree to which the host animal sees the new antigen as 'foreign'. Most published protocols give immunisation schedules in relation to physicochemical grouping without taking regard to these other factors as they are too variable to catalogue and they must therefore be seen as only a very general guide for an initial attempt.

4.1.2. The relevance of serum antibody titre

The serum titre elicited has undoubted relevance to the likelihood of specific hybridoma production. However, it relates primarily to the number of immunoglobulin producing cells and this in turn may not correlate with the number of cells in the chosen tissue suitable for fusion with the chosen partner to lead to immunoglobulin of the chosen specificity. In particular, rapidly dividing plasmablasts which do not themselves secrete large amounts of antibody have been shown to correlate with a high frequency of antigen specific hybridoma production. This is achieved by giving large doses of antigen intravenously without adjuvant on each of the 3–4 days preceeding the fusion using an animal which has been immunised by conventional means in the preceeding weeks (Stahli et al., 1980). All protocols recommend fusion 3–4 days after the final boost and it should be noted that the serum titre has not generally reached a maximum at this time.

4.1.3. Purity of antigen

One of the most misleading concepts which have grown up around monoclonal antibody technology is that there is no need to purify the antigen used for immunisation. While the concept is undoubtedly correct, in practice this is frequently unsatisfactory despite the spectacular early success in the case of interferon (Secher and Burke, 1980). In the great majority of cases, the major antigens dominate a fusion in the same way as they dominate a serum titre and some preliminary purification of minor antigens is highly desirable. While the sequential fusion technique in which the major antigen is adsorbed so that minor components may dominate the second fusion is a possible experimental approach (Fig. 4.1), it clearly consumes a very large amount of time. Immunisation with a pure protein from a fixed and stained bond of SDS–PAGE is reported to be a simple and successful procedure (Tracy et al., 1983).

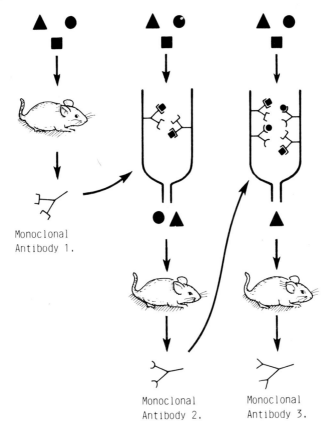

Fig. 4.1. Sequential fusion and purification of monoclonal antibodies from a complex mixture of antigens. The first fusion is dominated by the square antigen and the bulk of the monoclonal antibodies produced react with this. Before the second immunisation, the square antigen is removed from the mixture by the use of an affinity column of the monoclonal antibody produced by the first fusion reacting with it. The second experiment is dominated by antibodies to the round antigen and this is also removed by reaction with antibodies specific to it alone. The third and minor antigen can thus be used for the final immunisation to produce a panel of monoclonal antibodies specific to it, even although it was a minor (or less antigenic) component of the original mixture.

4.1.4. Tolerance, overimmunisation and underimmunisation

The general area of tolerance is a complex one and dealt with in greater depth in the major immunological textbooks referred to in the introduction to Chapter 1. For the purposes of hybridoma production, low zone tolerance which is achieved with continuous injections of subimmunogenic quantities of antigen is less likely to complicate a schedule as the amounts involved are very small. However, it should be noted that immunisation with very small amounts of a particularly scarce antigen in the hope of producing an immune response may yield poor results because of this phenomenon rather than for the more obvious reasons and such antigens are best used for in vitro immunisation. However, repeated injections of large amounts of antigen in order to increase the number of specific plasmablasts may lead to immune paralysis. In this condition the cell surface receptors may be blocked by antigen so that they cannot function normally or suppressor T cells may be activated. Soluble protein antigens are very much less likely to induce tolerance than particulate antigens.

There is some evidence (Oi et al., 1978) that over-immunisation can lead to the production of a smaller number of antigen positive clones. However, this is a single specific case with many other variables and cannot be taken as a general rule. Most antigens have multiple epitopes and may in addition have many impurities. Different amounts of immunisation may alter the frequencies of clones to any of the epitopes or to the impurities depending on the degree to which they are all immunogenic.

The most frequent practical problems which relate to this question usually arise from a situation where an animal has been boosted in preparation for a fusion with a valuable antigen and the fusion experiment is then cancelled because of other considerations. The animal can then be used for a fusion at a later date but the number and nature of antigen-specific hybridomas produced is unlikely to be the same as it would have been on the original date. It could of course be better.

It should be noted that the age of the animals used is another important variable and it is advisable to adhere fairly closely to the limits given. It is, in particular not usual to use any of the recommended mouse or rat strains over a year in age and preferable to use them very much younger.

4.1.5. The relationship between the immunising antigen and the antigen required

In general. the antigen used for immunisation is also the antigen to which the monoclonal antibody is required. However there may be exceptions to this situation. It should be noted, for example, that if a complex antigenic mixture cannot be avoided and suitable epitopes unique to the chosen antigen such as a unique peptide configuration or unusual carbohydrate combination are already known then it may be possible to consider immunisation with these components as 'artificial' antigens. Chemically synthesised peptides are attracting interest as vaccines and may have potential in monoclonal antibody work where the target epitope can be identified (Lerner, 1982).

For cell surface antigens it is possible to immunise animals with one cell type which contains the required antigen among many others and select with a different cell type which contains the same antigen but among a different group of competing antigens.

4.2. Immunisation schedules

Typical schedules are given in Protocols 4.1 and 4.2 together with notes on variations which have given satisfactory published results. The general surgical manipulations involved are given in Appendix 1. Before they are used, Section 4.1 should be read and interpreted for the antibody in question.

Protocol 4.1

Immunisation with soluble antigens, bacteria and viruses

(i) Inject a 6–10 week old mouse or rat of the selected genetic type (Chapter 3) with 1–10 µg of pure carbohydrate antigen, 10–50 µg of pure protein antigen and larger amounts of impure antigen, in general not exceeding 1000 µg. The antigen should be mixed with an equal amount of complete Freunds adjuvant. Mixing should be very thorough. Detailed procedures are available in Weir (1978). The simplest are a double hubbed needle joining two glass syringes or the injection of small aliquots of aqueous antigen with repeated vortexing but commercial emulsifiers may also be obtained. (Most sterile polypropylene syringes are not suitable for use with Freund's adjuvant.) The antigen is then introduced into the animal at several sites by subcutaneous or intradermal routes (Appendix 1). Intraperitoneal injection will also yield results but these may be of lower titre.

Note 1. The quantities suggested are very wide ranging but this reflects the very wide range successfully used in published work. The upper end of the scale will not necessarily lead to a higher frequency of antigen specific hybridomas. Smaller amounts have also frequently been successful and for some bacteria and viruses amounts of below 1 µg yield large numbers of hybridomas.

Note 2. Other adjuvants such as alum and/or *B. pertussis* (usually in the region of 10^9) are also used though less frequently.

(ii) After a further period of time in the range of 2–3 weeks inject the animal with a similar or larger dose intraperitoneally. After a further 4–6 days bleed the animal and check the titre using the assay which will be used for screening. If a positive titre in excess of 1 in 1000 is obtained a fusion experiment may be planned with reasonable optimism. If the titre is above 1 in 200 it may be planned. A lower titre is in general indicative of an inadequate response. This can either be because the assay is poorly planned and too insensitive (Chapter 2) or because the animal's response is poor.

Note 3. A poor response may possibly but not necessarily be improved by further immunisation of the animal. Too much complete adjuvant is, however, not recommended though it can be used once or twice again. If the animal still fails to respond it is best to start with a new animal varying the strain (Chapter 3), the amount used, the immunisation schedule, or the site of injection. To save time, most people faced with an apparently poor antigen vary several of these simultaneously. In vitro immunisation should also be considered (Section 4.3).

Note 4. It is quite possible to immunise an animal with a single dose and attempt a fusion four days later. While this has been quite successful for some antigens it is not a recommended general procedure. The titre of the animal will not reflect the number of antigen-positive cells suitable for fusion and there is no way of telling whether or not this was a suitable procedure until the first screen by which time much effort will have been expended. The procedures tend to select for IgM producing hybridomas.

(iii) If the animal shows a positive titre then it should be boosted intravenously with 4–5 times the original dose in saline or PBS 3–4 days before the fusion.

Note 5. For some antigens better responses are obtained if the animal is rested for a week or two before the boost and for most antigens a delay of several weeks at this stage is quite acceptable, so there is no need to hurry to plan the fusion after a good titre has been obtained. The 3–4-day period between boost and fusion is, however, critical and a longer time period will give poorer results.

Note 6. If the antigen is a stained band from an SDS gel then the homogenised mixture of gel and antigen may be injected.

Protocol 4.2

Immunisation with cellular antigens

(i) Inject a 4–12 week old mouse or rat with 1–5×10^7 cells in saline or PBS either intravenously or intraperitoneally. Do not use adjuvant.

Note 7. Published doses range from below 10^6 to above 10^7 so there is ample scope for variation. In particular if a primary tumour is the source of the cells, the numbers available may be limiting as the same cells are required for boosting and screening so the lower end of the range is usually employed and a panel of hybridomas is obtained without difficulty.

(ii) After 3 weeks reimmunise the animal with the same dose in the same manner. Bleed the animal after a further 4–6 days and check the titre using the assay that will be used for screening. As in protocol 4.2 a titre of 1 in 1000 or greater is an indication that successful fusion is likely, a titre of 1 in 200 that a successful fusion is possible. A titre of below 200 indicates that either the assay is at fault or too insensitive or the animal is not responding sufficiently well to the antigen. In this case see Protocol 4.1, Notes 3, 4 and 5.

(iii) If the titre is satisfactory, boost the animal with 4–5 times the original dose of cells 3–4 days before fusion. See Protocol 4.1, Note 5.

Note 8. It is obviously desirable to immunise the animal with the same batch of cells and this means that they must be stored between immunisations. The recommended storage procedures are either those for tissue culture cells in liquid nitrogen with 10% DMSO or at $-70°$ in buffer containing 0.25 M sucrose and 25% glycerol.

4.3. Immunisation in vitro

4.3.1. Rodent immunisation

Immunisation in vitro is frequently considered to be a technique only required in human hybridoma production. However there may be many situations in which it is also suitable for rodent antibody production. In particular, it is possible to produce antibodies to antigens suppressed in the normal response (Reading, 1982). It may also prove a more reproducible method of immunisation because of the comparative simplicity of the system and the possibility of maintaining defined concentrations of antigen. One major reported advantage is the fact that immunisation may be performed with nanogram quantities of antigen where milligram amounts may be required for in vivo immunisation (Pardue et al., 1983; Luben and Mohler, 1980). In addition, the immunisation procedure takes only a few days if speed is important and labile antigens may be used. A higher proportion of IgM-secreting hybridomas are generated in this technique though it is also possible to produce IgG secretors (Fig. 4.2).

Primary in vitro immunisation refers to an antigen to which the

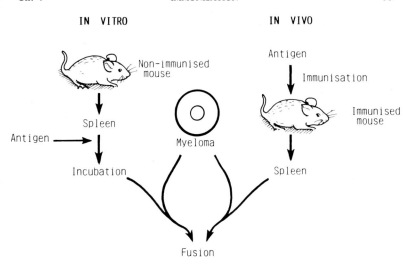

Fig. 4.2. A comparison of in vivo and in vitro immunisation.

animal has not been previously exposed. Secondary immunisation implies that the animal has been exposed to the antigen and may be expected to have memory cells for it. The distinction is not as clear as it may appear unless the animal has been kept in a highly controlled environment.

The procedure has little more complexity than the cell culture techniques required for the production of the antibodies themselves. For the rodent immunisations it is usual to use thymocyte-conditioned medium which contains lymphokines or other soluble factors which are thought to assist the in vitro immunisation. General cell culture procedures are given in Chapter 5 but the basic protocols are given here for convenience.

Protocol 4.3

Rodent in vitro immunisation
  (a) Preparation of thymocyte-conditioned medium

(i) Dissect out 5–10 thymus glands from 12–14-day old mice or rats of the same strain as will be used for the in vitro immunisation (see Appendix 1). It is important to use young animals as the thymus is very small in older ones. Rinse the animals in ethanol before dissection and do not rupture the oesophagus or the trachea as this will increase the chances of contamination. Rinse the organs well in serum-free RPMI.

(ii) Press the organs through a 50-mm mesh stainless steel screen into a 10-cm petri dish containing 5 ml serum free RPMI (see Section 5.2.3) using the plunger of a 10-ml disposable pipette. A domestic tea strainer is very suitable for this purpose. Alternatively the organs may be teased apart with two 21-G needles. Discard the capsule and further disperse the clumps of cells by sucking them twice up and down into a 10-ml sterile disposable syringe with a 21-G needle and then twice with a 25-G needle with moderate pressure.

(iii) Wash the cells twice in serum free RPMI by centrifugation at 1000 g in a 20-ml sterile universal and resuspension by gentle shaking pipetting with a 10-ml sterile pipette. Count the cells and resuspend them in RPMI supplemented with 5×10^{-5} M 2-mercaptoethanol and 20% foetal calf serum at a density of 5×10^6 cells/ml in a small plastic tissue culture flask. Incubate in a humidified CO_2 oven for 2–4 days.

(iv) Centrifuge to remove cell debris and filter the supernatant through a sterile 0.2-μm filter.

Note 1. This preparation is reported to be stable for many months when frozen at $-70\,°C$, so it is possible to undertake a large preparation and store the thymocyte conditioned medium in aliquots.

(b) Immunisation

(i) Prepare the antigen in RPMI + 10% foetal calf serum (FCS). The antigen must be sterile and if it is cellular must not be able to compete with the spleen cells for the nutrients in the medium. Soluble antigens may be filtered through a 0.2-μm nitrocellulose filter though some antigens tend to bind to the filter reducing the yield. Cellular and soluble antigens can be irradiated at 2500 rad with a ^{60}Co irradiator. Access to hospital X-ray machines is usually readily arranged if this is not available.

(ii) Dissect out the spleen from a 4–12-week-old mouse or rat of the same strain as the source of thymus. As above, rinse the animal in 70% ethanol and maintain the dissection as sterile as possible. Rinse the spleen in RPMI.

(iii) Using two 21-G needles tease the spleen cells free from the fibrous capsule in a 100-mm petri dish containing 5 ml serum-free RPMI. Disperse clumps of cells by sucking them twice up and down into a sterile syringe using a 21-G needle and twice with a 25-G needle using moderate pressure.

Note 1. It is also possible to prepare the spleen cells by pressing the spleen through a stainless steel mesh as in the thymocyte preparation. This is perfectly satisfactory but can result in a larger number of fibroblasts which tend to dominate the culture. Other techniques involve the gentle flushing out of the more mobile, rapidly dividing cells from the spleen and they are not recommended for this procedure since rapid cell division is yet to be induced.

(iv) Wash the spleen cells twice in 20-ml serum-free RPMI in a 20-ml universal container (see Table 5.2), centrifuging at 500 g for 5 min and resuspending with gentle shaking or pipetting with a 10-ml pipette.

(v) Resuspend the cells at a density of 5×10^6 cells/ml in the previously prepared RPMI + 10% FCS containing the antigen. The antigen concentration should be selected according to some of the considerations used for in vivo immunisation. In general, suitable concentrations for soluble antigens range over 0.05–5 µg/ml and cellular ones 10^5 to 10^6 cells/ml.

(vi) Add an equal volume of thymocyte conditioned medium to the culture. Incubate in a humidified CO_2 incubator for 4–5 days in a small tissue culture flask (20 ml) and then use the cells for fusion.

4.3.2. In vitro immunisation of human cells

Few detailed procedures for human work of this type have been published and the chances of success are very much lower than with the rodent system. In general, the same principles apply though stimulation with thymocyte-conditioned medium is not usually possible. In addition the human tissues available may differ. Most success is claimed with human tonsillar lymphocytes though spleens and peripheral blood lymphocytes are also used. Lymphocytes are generally further purified from other cells by centrifugation on Ficoll or Percoll (Section 7.3). The process is complex and to date there is little convincing data to suggest that true in vitro immunisation with a primary antigen has been achieved. This is particularly true where the chosen antigens are ovine or bovine red blood cells as allogeneic antigens can stimulate an in vitro response to these cells (Mori et al., 1981). Published data on protein antigens suggest that antigen concentration, T cell and possibly monocyte participation, and precise cell culture conditions are all vital factors (Lane et al., 1981) and it is not possible to give a consensus protocol at the moment.

4.3.3. In vitro immunisation with polyclonal activators

There are several well known polyclonal activators of the B cell response (Reading, 1982). In the rodent system there was much early interest in the use of lipopolysaccharide (LPS) (Andersson et al., 1979). LPS is known to stimulate a subpopulation of B cells to growth and antibody secretion. The stimulus may result in an increase in the number of actively dividing blast cells which are thought to lead to the production of a higher frequency of hybridomas. In principle, the likelihood of obtaining a specific hybridoma is thus increased. There is some evidence that a better response may be obtained by preincubation of the lymphocytes before LPS treatment (Ilfeld et al., 1981). LPS concentrations in the region of 50 µg/ml are used / 5×10^5 cells and the stimulation is normally performed over a period of 3–5 days. LPS preparations are very variable and each one must be tested for the optimal response. There have been some claims that the combination of antigen and LPS lead to an enhanced specific response and if in vitro immunisation with antigen alone fails to produce suitable hybridomas it is possible to attempt this approach. Poke weed mitogen (PWM) has also been claimed to enhance the response in human fusions (Warenius et al., 1983).

4.4. Isotype enrichment

4.4.1. Requirements for specific isotypes

Most laboratories do not set out to make hybridomas with any specific isotype requirement. There are however situations in which a specific requirement is dictated by the projected use of the monoclonal antibody. For example an IgG may be preferable to an IgM for therapeutic use because of its smaller size leading to greater tissue access. For other purposes a complement fixing IgM may be preferred. IgA antibodies provide host defence against mucosal pathogens and are sought in the study of this type of immunity and IgE antibodies are useful in studies on hypersensitivity. One obvious method of selecting a specific isotype is by assay (Chapter 2) with a second antibody directed towards a specific heavy chain. In the case of IgM and the IgG family this is a fairly acceptable procedure. However, IgA and IgE hybridomas are rare and in the case of IgA procedures have been developed to increase the frequency of production. The Fluorescence Activated Cell Sorter (Section 6.4) may also be used to select the correct isotype.

4.4.2. Enrichment for IgM

In vitro immunisation is a technique particularly suited to IgM production. If the immunisation is carried out in vivo for only 2–3 days the majority of the hybridomas are IgM. If it is carried out for longer the proportion of IgG rises to 50%. If, however, in vivo immunisation is employed then a single large dose of antigen 3–4 days before fusion also leads mainly to IgM producing hybridomas. In the case of the human system, transformation of lymphocytes with Epstein Barr virus (Chapter 6) prior to fusion also leads to a dominance of IgM-producing cells used in the subsequent fusion (Komisar et al., 1982).

It should be noted that in general IgM-producing hybridomas synthesise antibodies of lower affinity than IgG-producing hybridomas (Rodwell et al., 1983).

4.4.3. Enrichment for IgA production

The simplest method of immunising to produce IgA-specific hybridomas is by altering the immunisation route in vivo and administering the antigen by gastric intubation (Colwell et al., 1982) and subsequently carrying out a normal fusion using spleen cells from the immunised animal. A different method involves conventional immunisation of the animal followed by a fusion with the gut associated lymphoid tissue (Peyer's patch and mesenteric lymph node). A third method involves the adoptive transfer of cells from the gut associated lymphoid tissue (Peyer's patch and mesenteric lymph node) (Komisar et al., 1982).

4.4.4. Enrichment for IgE production

Freunds adjuvant is not suitable for IgE production and alum is recommended. In addition, adoptive transfer techniques are usually required (Tung, 1983).

CHAPTER 5

Cell culture requirements for hybridomas

5.1. Introduction

Cell culture is a complex process with many variables. An earlier volume in this series deals with general culture procedures in greater detail (Adams, 1980). This chapter is addressed to cell culture requirements specifically for hybridoma production.

5.2. Basic requirements

The basic requirements for cell culture are tabulated and costed in Table 5.1. In principle, it is quite possible to produce hybridomas in a general research laboratory equipped with a sterile hood and a carbon dioxide incubator. In practice it is, however, very useful to have a laboratory or an area of a laboratory set aside for hybridoma work and it is particularly advisable not to share sterile hoods and incubators with a large number of people whose technique may not be of the fairly high standards required.

It is essential to have an inverted microscope of reasonable quality to monitor the cells and, in particular, the appearance of the clones. A small bench centrifuge which need not be refrigerated for the great majority of the work is also necessary. While most solutions may be sterilised in a domestic pressure cooker, an autoclave for larger amounts is also strongly advised. If glassware etc. such as pipettes are to be sterilised, an autoclave is essential. However, sterile disposable pipettes may be purchased at higher overall running cost.

TABLE 5.1

Essential hardware for hybridoma production

Item	Suppliers	Typical cost (1983 U.K.)
Vertical laminar air flow hood with ultraviolet light	Flow Laboratories	£1700.00
Water jacketed carbon dioxide incubator	Flow Laboratories	£2600.00
Inverted microscope	Olympus CK	£ 750.00
Carbon dioxide regulators and valves	Distillers Company Ltd. (U.K. only)	£ 35.00 each
Liquid nitrogen storage vat	Various	Variable
(a) Domestic pressure cooker *or* (b) Autoclave	Various	(a) £ 25.00 (b) £4800.00
8 channel variable multipipettes (5–50 µl and 50–200 µl)	Flow Laboratories	£ 230.00 each

The list of suppliers given is obviously very limited and no commercial company is deliberately favoured. Firms which have branches in both the U.S.A. and Europe are noted in particular. In almost all cases a local supplier may be superior. Useful people to consult apart from other research laboratories which undertake tissue culture are hospitals which are particularly knowledgeable about supplies of gas cylinders and valves among other items. Cell culture is a growth area and many small local firms may supply all items on Table 5.1 at much reduced rates.

It is assumed that other essential items such as a haemocytometer for counting cells, automatic pipettes for the range 10–100 µl and refrigerators and freezers are already available. However, again a separate supply for the hybridoma work is invaluable.

5.2.1. Additional useful items

Multipipettes are particularly useful for sampling if the assay system involves a microelisa plate of the same dimensions. These may be obtained in 4, 8 or 12 channel varieties. An automatic pipetting device saves much time and is relatively inexpensive. A box for autoclaving the tips of automatic pipettes is extremely useful.

5.2.2. Plastic ware

Table 5.2 gives a list of plasticware with typical costs. Costar plates of both sizes (96 and 24 well) are necessary. These particular plates are recommended because of the independent structure of each well minimising the possibility of transfer of contaminants between wells. The other requirements are petri dishes, plastic flasks of all three main sizes, pipettes and tips, and large numbers of sterile 20-ml universal containers. Protective gloves and autoclave bags are not included but often required. Glass, reusable pipettes with plugged cotton wool tips may also be used and these are undoubtedly cheaper.

TABLE 5.2
Essential plasticware for hybridoma production

Item	Typical annual use per operator (highly variable)	Supplier	Typical cost (1984, U.K.)
96-well plates	50–100 plates	COSTAR	£50/48 plates
24-well plates	50–100 plates	COSTAR	£75/100 plates
1-ml sterile pipettes	400–600	COSTAR	£20/200 pipettes
5-ml sterile pipettes	400–600	COSTAR	£35/200 pipettes
10-ml sterile pipettes	400–600	COSTAR	£35/200 pipettes
Petri dishes (60 mm)	200	COSTAR	£55/200 dishes
Universal containers (20 ml)	600	NUNC	£20/300 containers
25-cm^2 tissue culture flasks	100	NUNC	£45/160 flasks
80-cm^2 culture flasks	50	NUNC	£26/50 flasks
175-cm^2 tissue culture flasks	20	NUNC	£30/32 flasks
Ampoules for liquid nitrogen preservation	200	NUNC	£50/500 ampoules

5.2.3. Media

Two main types of media are used at the moment for hybridoma production. These are Dulbecco's Modification of Eagles Medium (DMEM) and Rosewell Park Memorial Institute (RPMI) medium. Iscove's modification of DMEM (Section 5.2.4) is also successful though it is used less frequently. Throughout this book RPMI is the medium specificied. However, in nearly all cases DMEM will perform equally well. There are differences in the media, for example basic DMEM has pyruvate where RPMI does not and has more bicarbonate buffer so is better if it has to sit around in the absence of CO_2. Formulations and suppliers are given in the manufacturer's catalogues (Flow; Gibco; Appendix 2). Liquid medium is usually supplied without glutamine because of its comparative instability in aqueous solution and it must be added to a level of 2 mM. Powdered medium is usually purchased with glutamine already present. Various protocols throughout the years recommend the addition of pyruvate at 1 mM, glycine at up to 100 mM and 2-mercaptoethanol at 50 μM. None of these are necessary for successful hybridoma production but they can do little harm. Mercaptoethanol, is however still thought to be necessary for in vitro immunisation (Chapter 4). Media are made up in double distilled water, sterilised by filtration through 0.2-μm membranes, and usually stored in 500–1000 ml aliquots for up to 6 weeks. Both main recommended media are bicarbonate buffered with phenol red indicator. The correct colour for medium is bright orange indicating a pH of 7.2. Yellow medium is acid and is found where strong growth has occurred.

5.2.4. Sera

Foetal calf serum (FCS) is used in nearly all hybridoma work. This can be obtained from most suppliers of tissue-culture equipment (Flow, Gibco, see Appendix 2). Most reputable suppliers are prepared to send several samples from different batches for the laboratory to test and an order can then be placed for the most suitable. Ideally, the serum should be tested by determining the cloning efficiency of an established hybridoma. However, this is clearly a chicken and egg situation and it may be adequately tested on the parent cell line. FCS is usually obtained in sterile 100-ml aliquots. These are heated to inactivate complement at 56° for 30 min. The serum is kept frozen at −20°. FCS is particularly useful for hybridoma work because of the low level of contaminating immunoglobulin. However, different batches can have up to 1.3 mg/ml bovine IgG which may be comparable to or greater than the levels of hybridoma secreted antibody (Underwood et al., 1983). Newborn calf serum is sometimes substituted and is generally cheaper but less good. Horse and rabbit serum are also sometimes used. However, these will be contaminated with immunoglobulins. Serum-free medium is becoming increasingly widely used in many laboratories and Iscove and Melchers (1978) have developed a medium in which B lymphocytes may be cultured using enriched DMEM, albumin, transferrin and lecithin (Barnes and Sato, 1980). More recently, Murakami et al. (1982) have used a serum-free medium based on RPMI with insulin as well as the other additives for specific use with mouse hybridomas. There is no doubt that serum-free medium will be much used in the future because of its clearly reproducible characteristics but it is infrequently used for hybridoma work at the moment.

5.2.5. Antibiotics

The basic antibiotics used in hybridoma production are penicillin and streptomycin (P/S). The former inhibits the growth of most gram-positive bacteria and the latter the growth of most gram-negative ones. Penicillin and streptomycin preparations may be obtained from a variety of suppliers such as Flow and Gibco (Appendix 2). They are usually made up in × 100 stock solutions containing 10^7 units of sodium benzyl penicillin and 10 g of streptomycin sulphate per litre. This is filter-sterilised through 0.2-μm membranes, and stored in 20-ml aliquots at −20°. Prepared stock solutions may be purchased from all major tissue-culture suppliers. It is not advisable to propagate stock cell lines continuously in P/S in case resistant strains arise. Some laboratories use Fungizone (Amphotericin B) at 2.5 μg/ml medium routinely, others only where contamination has occurred.

5.2.6. Other chemicals

The components of HAT solution previously mentioned in Chapter 3 are further discussed in Chapter 6. They may be obtained from most of the main fine chemical companies and the supplier does not seem to be a critical factor (Appendix 2). Dimethyl sulphoxide is definitely required for freezing and thawing of cells and some laboratories incorporate it in the fusion procedure. It may be sterilised by autoclaving or filtration. A strong disinfectant such as chloros is also necessary.

5.3. Basic cell-culture techniques

Many cell-culture techniques are not covered in this volume but the basic ones necessary for simple hybridoma work are given in detail. More elaborate techniques are covered by Adams (1980).

5.3.1. General sterile technique

While all tissue culture requires good sterile technique, hybridoma production requires a particularly high standard because of the number of manipulations involved in feeding and sampling. The personnel involved should have a high standard of hygiene with clean hair, beards, clothes and fingernails. They should not drink beer and especially real ale and not make bread in the 24 h before fusion or cloning are carried out. Ideally hands should be well washed and swabbed in 70% ethanol before they enter the hood. The hood should be kept scrupulously clean and swabbed down with 70% ethanol. Bunsen burners are not generally used in vertical flow hoods and can indeed be dangerous in an atmosphere of ethanol. All bottles of medium etc. should be wiped and swabbed at the stoppers with 70% ethanol before being put into the hood. The 37° water bath in which they are warmed should be cleaned and disinfected regularly. The incubator should be inspected regularly and cleaned every 2–3 months with disinfectant. No old cultures with spent medium should be allowed to remain in it and no arms covered in dirty woollen sweaters should be allowed to reach into it. All solutions and glassware should, of course, be sterilised by autoclaving or filtration.

The actual experimental material may also be a source of contamination. Animals should not be handled in the sterile hood, even if they have been swabbed with ethanol. Every cell line received from an outside laboratory should be checked for mycoplasma. Human tissues can be another source of mycoplasma and should be handled in a separate hood where possible.

It will be evident from the above that shared equipment can pose problems. The standard of sterility is effectively as high as that of the least hygienic operator. In a large group it is sensible to have very firm cleaning and inspection rotas and if possible to train any new member of the group with extreme care and on facilities outwith the main hybridoma equipment.

5.3.2. Complete medium

Basic medium is usually made up in 100–500-ml aliquots. For 100-ml batch at 10% fetal calf serum, 90 ml of RPMI with glutamine and combined with 10 ml FCS and 1 ml stock solution of P/S. This medium can be used for the propagation of the parent line and is also adequate for growth of the cells after fusion and limiting dilution cloning. However, some laboratories prefer to use 20% FCS at early stages after fusion and for cloning. A fully established hybridoma and healthy parent cell line will also grow well in 5% FCS. There is often some confusion where the term 'medium' is used in protocols. In this book 'medium' refers to RPMI alone while 'complete medium' refers to RPMI + P/S + serum. The actual serum concentration is usually specified.

5.3.3. Freezing and thawing of cells

This procedure is obviously important in hybridoma work. Freezing of cells which have not been cloned after the primary fusion is not always successful, presumably because of overgrowth by non-producing cells. However the parent myeloma and established hybridomas can be stored with little difficulty. The cells are centrifuged and resuspended at $5-10 \times 10^6$ cells/ml in 70% RPMI + 20% FCS + 10% DMSO. 1.5-ml aliquots of this suspension are then pipetted into plastic storage ampoules and frozen slowly at $-70°$ in a plastic ampoule placed in a polystyrene box for at least 12 h. The ampoules are then transferred to liquid nitrogen. Controlled cooling equipment is now commercially available (Cryotech or Cryoson) and the recommended freezing rate is $1°C/min$. Some laboratories prefer to freeze cells in 50% FCS (+ 40% RPMI + 10% DMSO) and some in 90% FCS + 10% DMSO. Wells et al. (1983) have reported a procedure for freezing cells in tissue culture plates.

Thawing in contrast is done speedily. The ampoule is thawed in a 37° water bath and the contents are transferred to a small plastic flask containing 10 ml of complete medium (10% FCS). If smaller numbers of cells have been frozen they should be transferred to a 2-ml well of a 24-well Costar plate and if very small numbers of cells have been frozen feeders are advisable. Only 10–20% of the cells will recover from freezing.

5.3.4. Cell counting and viability checks

Cell counting is by the use of the Neubauer haemocytometer or counting chamber. These vary slightly but each one is supplied with exact specifications and amplification factors. In order to check viability the cells are stained with a dye which differentiates dead from live cells. Typical dyes are trypan blue (0.2 g/l in 0.15 M NaCl), and eosin (0.05 g/l in 0.15 M NaCl) both of which stain dead cells. Nigrosine (0.2%) is also used. These checks are particularly important before fusion where high viability is required (Chapter 6).

5.4. Contamination

Contamination is best avoided totally by the precautions given in Section 5.3. If it occurs, whatever the source, the culture is best removed and autoclaved without opening immediately. Any attempt to rescue a contaminated culture may put all the other cultures in the laboratory at risk. For this reason it is recommended that a vital culture of which there are no spare stocks be frozen, if there are enough cells, and split and kept in separate incubators and fed with separate batches of medium until enough cells have been obtained for freezing and further propagation.

There is no doubt that the failure of most hybridoma experiments is due to contamination and most of this is probably mycoplasma. Fungal and bacterial contamination may also occur but are more easily avoided.

5.4.1. Bacterial contamination

Bacterial contamination is very readily detected. The medium becomes acid and microscopic examination shows bacteria rather than cells. The use of penicillin and streptomycin minimises bacterial contamination. However resistant strains of bacteria can develop in the stock lines and cultures. For this reason the continual propagation of these in culture is not advised and batches should be grown, frozen in liquid nitrogen and thawed when required. This is also true of established hybridoma lines. If bacterial contamination does in fact develop the following order of priorities should be adopted.

If the contamination is in a stock culture of which there are plenty frozen supplies, then it should be disposed off immediately without opening of the flask or plate top. Autoclave the entire preparation and bring fresh cells up from liquid nitrogen.

If the contamination is in a vital cell line in a flask and there are no spare supplies, it is possible to use a third antibiotic such as gentamycin (200 µg/ml) which affects both gram-positive and -negative bacteria. The cells should be centrifuged and placed in fresh medium with the new antibiotic. If the cells are to be put back in culture in a shared incubator it is advisable to use a sealed gassed box and to warn other users.

If the contamination is in a Costar plate in a fusion which has several plates, the plate is best autoclaved without opening. However, if the contamination is only in a few wells and the plate is considered vital, it is possible to aspirate the contents of the well and wash it several times with chloros or other strong disinfectant. Some laboratories use 5 N NaOH for this purpose.

5.4.2. Fungal contamination

Fungal contamination tends to vary much with laboratory environment and is common in old buildings with inefficient air-conditioning systems. The fungus grows fast and is frequently not detected until it shows as a fluffy ball on top of the culture. At this stage it is very infectious. Do not open the bottle or Costar plate but autoclave it immediately. Further contamination may be avoided by the use of fungizone (Amphotericin B 2.5 µg/ml medium, available made up from Flow or Gibco). Note that fungizone is only stable for 3–4 days in water and bad fungal contamination necessitates regular medium changes which is not good for the emerging clones.

5.4.3. Contamination with mycoplasma

Bad mycoplasma contamination can lead to a laboratory having no successful fusions for a period of months. Preventive measures are therefore the most effective. As mentioned in Section 5.3 the operators selected for the hybridoma work must have a high standard of cleanliness, particularly in hands and hair. No cell line obtained from another source should be grown in the laboratory without first being checked for mycoplasma. Human tissues, particularly tonsil and lung, should be handled in a separate hood where possible.

Mycoplasma are small prokaryotes without a cell wall which grow in and around the cytoplasm of the mammalian cells which they have infected. Their biology is reviewed by Smith (1971). They are also known as PPLO (pleuropneumonia-like organisms). There are a wide variety of mycoplasma types and not all cause cell death. Most retard growth rate. Their nutritional requirements are such that they can deplete the culture medium of certain nutrients in a highly selective manner and their undoubtedly disastrous effects on cell-fusion experiments are attributed to the fact that they cleave thymidine to its component sugar and base very efficiently thus making selective HAT medium ineffective.

There are several tests for mycoplasma but the most effective is probably the fluorescent method utilising either Hoechst 33258 (0.05 μg/ml) (Hilwig and Gropp, 1972) or 4,6-diamidino-2-phenylindole (0.1 μg/ml) (Russel et al., 1975). These dyes bind to DNA. Cytoplasmic fluorescence indicates the presence of mycoplasma. The Hoechst stain is generally used on fixed cells (ethanol–acetic acid 3:1) but the DAPI can be used with unfixed cells. Complete commercial kits using the Hoechst stain may be purchased from Flow laboratories and a commercial kit which utilises DAPI may be purchased from Bioassay. Control cells used should include cells known to be mycoplasma-free and it is helpful to stain for a variety of times so that the cytoplasmic fluorescence may be detected before it is overshadowed by the nuclear fluorescence. Conventional staining methods using orcein (Fogh and Fogh, 1968) and autoradiography (Nardone et al., 1965) may also be used. Many commercial tissue-culture companies will test cells for mycoplasma at reasonable cost. Biological tests such as uridine uptake may also be used. Fluorescent staining is unsuitable for cell lines such as B95-8 which secrete a virus (Section 3.6.4).

If the parent cell lines have mycoplasma they should all be autoclaved, the hood and incubator should be cleaned with detergent, and new myeloma lines should be obtained from a fresh source. Even then, mycoplasma may persist so regular checks are advisable with the fresh material. If it is not possible to obtain fresh parent lines then kanomycin (100 μg/ml) (Fogh and Hacker, 1960), tylocine (sometimes called tylosin; 10–50 μg/ml) or lincomycin and vanomycin (Adams, 1980) have been reported to be able to prevent the growth of at least some species. Treatment of the cells at elevated temperatures has also been reported to be useful (Pollock and Kenny, 1963). A detailed procedure recommended by Schimmelpfeng et al. (1980) involves the incubation of small numbers of myeloma cells with activated mouse peritoneal macrophages in complete medium in a well of a 24-well Costar plate in the presence of 100 µg/ml lincomycin and 100 µg/ml tylocine for 7 days. An alternative procedure from Marcus et al. (1980) utilises the ability of mycoplasma to use bases rather than nucleosides better than the parent cell and also their high AT base content. The cells are incubated with 5-bromouracil which is preferentially incorporated into the mycoplasma DNA and then with Hoechst 33258. Irradiation of the subsequent complex causes preferential damage to the myco-plasma DNA. One of the best reported methods however, with myelomas or hybridomas, is to passage them through the ascitic fluid of a mouse or rat (see Chapter 9).

5.4.4. Contamination with viruses

Viral contamination is not usually a serious problem in hybridoma work. However, if human lymphocytes are used there is a high probability that they will have latent Epstein Barr (EB) virus and will become transformed in culture, especially in the absence of T lympho-cytes toxic to this virus. Many reported human fusions are not in fact fusions but transformations. (This may be a very suitable method for 'monoclonal antibody' production but may also not be what was intended.) Lymphocyte donors are tested for antibody to the viral capsid antigen (VCA) by use of the cell line P3 HR1 which secretes non-transforming EB. The cells are suspended at 2×10^6 cells/ml, placed on a slide, air-dried and acetone fixed for 10 min. A large batch may then be made and stored at $-70°$. Serum samples are then tested in doubling dilutions of PBS. One drop is added to each slide which is incubated in a humidified box at 37° for 1 h, washed, reacted with fluorescent labelled anti-human IgG (Miles) diluted 1/20 in PBS, washed again and covered with PBS + 10% glycerol. Both a positive and negative control sample are helpful in this test. Transformed cells can also be detected by their shape (Chapter 7) and by the fact that the resultant monoclonal antibody producing cell will only have one heavy and one light chain unlike most human hybridomas (Chapter 10).

5.4.5. Contamination with yeast

Contamination with yeast is comparatively rare. Usually it occurs with operators who drink beer or ale or bake bread but sometimes it occurs with no obvious source of contamination. The use of antifungal agents such as fungizone (Amphotericin B, 2.5 µg/ml) or nystatin (50 µg/ml) should guard against both yeast contamination as well. As before, the culture is best autoclaved and started afresh.

5.5. Feeder cells

Feeder cells or conditioned medium of some sort are absolutely essential for cloning of hybridomas. They are not necessary immediately after the fusion step but may help in situations where low cell densities are employed. If phagocytic cells such as macrophages and monocytes are used they can perform a helpful service in cleaning up the debris of dead cells always found after aminopterin treatment. The few comparative studies performed are not comprehensive and for the rodent system at least, most feeder systems will work. There are in fact three basic philosophies of feeding. The first is to use a (usually) allogeneic cell type with a limited lifetime which will nourish the emerging hybridomas and then die itself. The second is to use irradiated cells which grow well in themselves and may consequently be expected to have extra useful growth factors but are crippled by the irradiation so cannot divide and dominate the culture. The third is to use conditioned medium in which cells have been actively grown without irradiation for a period of 2–3 weeks. The cells are then removed and only the medium is used for feeding. This will permit the use of all the soluble growth factors (for example lymphokines from T cells) but gives the emerging hybridomas no cell contact which may be of value at low density. If feeders are to be used in the actual fusion, then the laying down of feeders on the day before fusion is recommended here. It is not necessary but it is convenient for the operator and gives the feeders time to establish.

5.5.1. Mouse feeder cells. Spleen cells

Spleen cells are convenient to use as feeders. The spleen is the organ of choice for the fusion and therefore the operator is used to dissecting and preparing spleen cells. Cells should be from the same strain of animal as that used in the fusion though successful fusions have been reported with xenogenic feeders. The procedure for preparing feeders is given in Protocol 5.1.

Protocol 5.1
Spleen feeder cell preparation
(i) Make up 100-ml complete medium at 10% FCS. Lay out sterile dissecting instruments, 100 ml RPMI, 100 ml complete medium, 2 × 6-cm petri dishes, 2 × 21-G needles and 2 × 25-G needles, 2 × 10-ml disposable syringes, at least five sterile 20-ml universal tubes, an eppendorf tube containing 0.3 ml 0.9% ammonium chloride, a stock of 5- and 10-ml pipettes, micropipettes capable of 0.1–0.5 ml delivery with sterile tips, and 4 × 96-well (or 24-well Costar plates).

(ii) Kill an 8–12-week-old mouse of the same genetic strain as the mouse used for the fusion. *DO NOT DO THIS IN THE STERILE HOOD*. Wash the mouse in 70% ethanol and remove the spleen (Appendix 1) using sterilised instruments. Transfer the spleen to a sterile universal tube containing RPMI and transfer this to the sterile hood. Wash the spleen twice with serum free RPMI and dissect off any fatty tissue with sterile instruments.

(iii) Put the spleen into a 6-cm petri dish containing 5 ml RPMI. Gently tease the spleen cells apart from the capsule using the two 21-G needles to break up clumps.

Draw the spleen cell suspension into a 10-ml sterile pipette using a 21-G needle and pipette it out again into a fresh petri dish. Repeat once with a 21-G needle and twice with a 25-G needle. Use only moderate pressure. Pipette the spleen cells direct from the syringe into a universal tube and centrifuge for 5 min at 500 g.

(iv) Wash the spleen cells twice with RPMI centrifuging as before and gently tapping the pellet to resuspend. If the technique is not familiar, count the spleen cells by pipetting a 0.05-ml aliquot into the eppendorf tube containing the 0.3 ml of ammonium chloride as this will help the cells to swell and lyse erythrocytes. Each mouse spleen should have about 10^8 cells and this figure can be assumed to save time.

(v) Resuspend the cells in 5 ml complete medium and dilute aliquots to 10^6 cells/ml in complete medium. Plate out on 96-well Costar plates at 0.1 ml $(1 \times 10^5$ cells)/well on 96-well Costar plates or 0.5 ml $(5 \times 10^5$ cells)/well on 24-well Costar plates. Incubate in the humidified incubator.

Note. The choice of 96- or 24-well Costar plates is further discussed in Section 6.4. In general it is best to start with 24-well ones and if fusions are successful move to 96-well ones.

5.5.2. Mouse feeders. Macrophages

Macrophages are probably the best feeders to use for hybridoma production immediately after fusion as they are active phagocytes. In the week after a fusion there is massive cell death of the parent myeloma line due to the aminopterin and emerging clones may be very difficult to see. Macrophages remove much of the debris. This function is not required in subcloning to the same extent but macrophages also provide a suitable environment in this situation.

Protocol 5.2

Macrophage feeder preparation

(i) Make up 100 ml complete medium + 10% FCS. Lay out complete medium, 100 ml PBS, two 10-ml syringes, two 21-G needles, several 20-ml universal containers, several sterile 5- and 10-ml pipettes, micropipettes capable of delivering 0.1–0.5 ml sterile tips and 4 × 96-well or 24-well Costar plates.

(ii) Kill an 8–12 week old mouse of the same strain as that to be used for the fusion. Prepare the macrophages according to Appendix 1. Keep the cells cool to avoid the tendency of macrophages to clump. Centrifuge at 500 g for 5 min, wash with PBS twice with centrifugation and count. Each mouse should yield 4×10^6 macrophages.

(iii) Resuspend in 40 ml complete medium + P/S and plate out at 0.1 ml (10^4 cells)/well in 96-well Costar plates or 0.5 ml (5×10^4 cells)/well in 24-well Costar plates. Incubate in a humidified incubator.

Note. Activated macrophages may be obtained by intraperitoneal injection of 1 ml 10% sodium thioglycollate four days before sacrificing the animal. Activated macrophages are also common in older animals. Some groups do not recommend these as they are too active and may cause hybridoma damage. They are, however, used for procedures such as mycoplasma elimination (Section 5.4.3).

5.5.3. Mouse feeders. Blood

Blood is not widely used as a feeder but appears to work well. One reported advantage is that emerging clones are readily viewed against the erythrocyte background. It may be obtained by the methods outlined in Appendix 1 (Section A.1.6.2.4). It is usually possible to obtain at least 1 ml of blood from a mouse and this is used as a concentration of 1% v/v in complete medium.

5.5.4. Other mouse feeders

Allogeneic or xenogeneic thymocytes are occasionally employed as feeders for cloning at 10^5/well in 96-well plates (Lernhardt et al., 1978; Oi and Herzenberg, 1980). These are in general harder to obtain. A 2–3-week-old mouse yields only 5×10^6 cells so that for extensive subcloning several mice may be required. Older mice have thymuses which are as large physically but less active biologically. In using thymocytes, an active T cell response may be generated and the lymphokines released may affect the subcloning. (For example thymocyte conditioned medium is used for in vitro immunisation, Chapter 4, Protocol 4.3.) Thymocytes are generally regarded as good but inconvenient feeders and may be employed in situations in which other feeder systems fail.

Conditioned medium from almost any actively growing mouse cell line may also be used. The data on the success of such procedures are sparse. Pintus et al. (1983) have reported that endothelial cell growth supernatant from bovine neural tissue is superior to macrophages and has the advantage of being available commercially, from Collaborative Research Inc., Waltham, MD.

5.5.5. Human feeder cells for human hybridomas

The easiest human feeders to obtain are peripheral blood mononuclear (PBL) cells and a procedure for the preparation of these is given in Protocol 5.3. They should be irradiated before use. The use of fresh human blood obtained from a laboratory donor is recommended but in the U.K. it is also possible to obtain buffycoats from the local blood transfusion service for bona fide medical research.

Protocol 5.3
Preparation of human PBL feeders

(i) Prepare a solution of Ficoll (Pharmacia). Lay out at least 8 sterile 20-ml universal containers, RPMI alone and complete medium (10% FCS + P/S) and a selection of sterile 10-ml pipettes.

(ii) Withdraw 20 ml fresh blood from a donor. Dilute the blood 1 in 2 in RPMI.

(iii) Layer the blood over an equal volume of Ficoll in sterile 20-ml universal containers. Centrifuge at 500 g for 15 min.

(iv) The red blood cells and polymorphs will centrifuge to the bottom of the tube. The peripheral blood mononuclear cells which include B and T lymphocytes and monocytes will remain at the interface. Remove the interfacial layer and dilute with an equal volume of RPMI. Centrifuge at 500 g for 5 min.

(v) Resuspend the cell pellet in complete medium, count and adjust to 3×10^6 cells/ml. There should be in the region of 3×10^7 cells so the total volume should be of the order of 10 ml.

(vi) Irradiate at 2000 R. Dilute in complete medium and plate out at 5×10^4 cells/well in 0.1 ml in flat bottomed 96-well Costar plates or 10^5 cells/ml in round bottomed Costar plates.

The best feeders for the rodent system are probably macrophages because of their phagocytic properties. On this basis, the best human feeders may well be monocytes and a procedure for the production of enriched monocytes is given by Brodin et al. (1983). It is interesting to note that they have also found mouse thymocytes to be efficient feeders for human hybridomas.

Many other feeder sytems are available such as irradiated human foetal fibroblasts (Kozbor and Roder, 1981) or cord blood. These are not readily obtained. Astaldi et al. (1980) recommend a complex culture supernatant from human endothelial cells isolated from umbilical cord veins for mouse–mouse hybridomas claiming that it can substitute totally for cells even at the high dilutions required in cloning. For human–mouse systems, the same group recommend the endothelial cells themselves (Astaldi et al., 1982).

5.5.6. Mouse feeder cells for human hybridomas

Where a human–mouse fusion has been performed and in many human–human fusions, the resultant clones are more mouse than human and mouse feeders may be used. For example Cote et al. (1983) used mouse peritoneal cells which are largely macrophages for both mouse–human and human–human hybrids. It is also possible to grow human cells on normal or irradiated mouse feeders other than the thymocytes. Edwards et al. (1982) use mouse peritoneal macrophages for the H-My2 human cell line with satisfactory results.

The area of human fusions is fast expanding and complex. The suggested practice for the moment is to use either mouse macrophages, or human PBLs. If these fail it is worth trying mouse thymus cells and watching the current literature closely. It is also worth remembering that the recommended feeders do undoubtedly work in some laboratories and it is probably better to improve tissue-culture technique or extend the range of the subcloning rather than to spend a large amount of time obtaining a complex feeder preparation.

CHAPTER 6

Fusion procedures

6.1. The use of polyethylene glycol

6.1.1. Introduction

While early experiments in cell fusion were performed with enveloped viruses such as Sendai virus (Harris and Watkins, 1965), nearly all fusions designed to produce hybridomas are now performed with chemical fusogens and polyethylene glycol (PEG) (Fig. 6.1) is the major chemical used. Early fusions also involved mammalian cells which were attached to the glass or plasticware and fusions in suspension require slightly different conditions (Gefter et al., 1977). The mechanism of fusion is complex, involving cell agglutination, membrane fusion, and cell swelling and the optimal environmental conditions for the three processes are frequently at variance (Knutton and Pasternak, 1979). It is interesting to note the wide variation in concentration and molecular weight and particular in the medium in which the PEG is made up which have all been used for successful hybridoma production. In addition, there are a large number of other chemicals which will also promote cell fusion (Klebe and Mancuso, 1981).

$$HO(CH_2CH_2O)_n CH_2CH_2OH$$

Fig. 6.1. The structure of polyethylene glycol (PEG).

6.1.2. Molecular weight

PEG may be obtained in the molecular weight range 200–20 000 (Fig. 6.1). It is toxic to cells and low molecular weight PEG is more toxic than high molecular weight PEG. Furthermore, the toxicity varies for each particular cell type. High molecular weight PEG is viscous and difficult to work with. Most successful fusions are performed with PEG in the molecular weight region 600–6000 (Davidson et al., 1976; Klebe and Mancuso, 1981). The supplier of the PEG is also considered to be a critical factor, and it may be relevant to note that the number stated on the supplier's bottle does not always refer to the exact molecular weight of the PEG. There is always a range of molecular weights rather than a single figure in each preparation. In view of the higher toxicity of the low molecular weight material, it is obviously important to obtain an undegraded preparation. Fazekas de St. Groth and Scheidegger (1980) have made a comparison of several suppliers and recommend Merck 4000 GK as the best PEG from the range tested. However, others have had very satisfactory results with material from Koch-Light and Serva. Our own laboratory has made very satisfactory hybridomas with material from BDH which is declared by some others to yield no fused cells at all.

6.1.3. Temperature and pH

Many published protocols suggest the use of PEG at 37°. This will do no harm but it is not necessary and is often inconvenient in a sterile hood though special heating blocks may be obtained. In a limited study, Klebe and Mancuso (1981) have shown that room temperature is superior to 37° and that the optimum pH is in the region of 7.5 though again the range is wide. Fazekas de St. Groth and Scheidegger (1980) show that room temperature is superior to 4°C. Room temperature and the use of medium (which is weakly buffered) are therefore in the recommended protocols.

6.1.4. Concentration

While the exact mechanisms of fusion are not fully understood, it is thought that the main function of the hydrophilic PEG is to occupy the 'physical free water' space leading to agglutination of the cells. This occurs at concentrations of PEG in the region of 40–50% and most fusions are performed within this range. There is, however, some variation of the optimum concentration with cell line (Gefter et al., 1977) and successful fusions can be performed at lower PEG concentrations such as 35% sometimes with a longer exposure time.

6.1.5. Other components of the PEG solution

Many fusions are undertaken using PEG in 15% DMSO as a result of the work of Norwood et al. (1976) who reported considerable enhancement of fusion frequencies of attached fibroblasts by addition of this reagent. The exact nature of the effect is not understood but may in some way relate to the distribution of water molecules between the various components during fusion. DMSO has not been fully tested for fusions in suspension although Fazekas de St. Groth and Scheidegger (1980) in a limited study concluded that it was only necessary where the addition of the fusion reagents was undertaken under suboptimal conditions. There is no doubt that DMSO is not necessary and its value is certainly dubious. It is not included in the protocols given in this Chapter.

A wide variety of buffers and reagents are used to dissolve the PEG. The most common is serum-free medium of the type employed in the fusion e.g. RPMI. However, phosphate-buffered saline (PBS) or Tris are also used. There is some confusion over the role of calcium ions which have been reported to be essential for fusion (Ahkong et al., 1973) and inhibitory to fusion (Klebe and Mancuso, 1981) and are in fact neither vital or inhibitory according to established procedures. As no systematic studies are published and most buffers work, the use of serum-free medium is recommended here. The refinement of adding 2 × medium to the autoclaved PEG is unnecessary. Lovborg

(1982) reports HEPES inhibitory to fusions but gives no data while Klebe and Mancuso (1981) report it to be the best among the buffers and media tested. Successful fusions can in fact be performed with PEG dissolved in sterile distilled water, although this is not recommended.

6.2. The components of HAT medium

There is happily less variability in the components of HAT medium and most fusion protocols utilise similar concentration ranges. Variation on concentrations is only applied under specific experimental conditions. Hypoxanthine is generally not toxic to cells and concentrations of 0.1 mM are used. Thymidine on the other hand can cause cessation of DNA synthesis at millimolar levels due to a feedback inhibition leading to a reduced pool size of dCTP. For this reason the concentration of thymidine is maintained at 0.016 mM. Thymidine inhibition is reversed by the use of deoxycytidine which allows the blockage to be bypassed and some protocols incorporate deoxycytidine for this reason. T cell hybridomas are exceptionally sensitive to thymidine by two orders of magnitude lower than most mammalian cultured cells and selection in the presence of deoxycytidine (Fox et al., 1980) or in 0.1 mM hypoxanthine with azaserine at 1 μg/ml is sometimes used under these conditions (Foung et al., 1982). Azaserine blocks the pathways of purine biosynthesis but not of pyrimidine biosynthesis. Thymidine deficiency is responsible for most of the difficulties encountered in attempts to fuse mycoplasma contaminated cells as many species of mycoplasma carry an enzyme which cleaves the base–sugar bond. Aminopterin inhibits metabolic pathways distinct from those involving nucleotide biosynthesis, notably the synthesis of some amino acids such as glycine and is therefore used at the mimimal effective dosage which is in the region of 0.4 μM. Some protocols incorporate additional glycine for this reason.

6.3. Selection of hybridomas by fluorescence activated cell sorting

The fluorescence activated cell sorter (FACS) is a very powerful tool for the isolation of hybridomas. The antigen is coupled to a fluorescent label and allowed to react with the fused cells. Hybridomas producing the appropriate antibodies may then be separated from the other components of the fusion mixture (Parks et al., 1979). The subject is reviewed by Dangl and Herzenberg (1982). The need for cloning is not totally removed since any fusion may generate a variety of hybridomas of different idiotype but much of the labour or selection and cloning is removed. In principal, it is possible to deflect a single desired hybridoma cell into a tissue culture well and clone it from the start and many clones with varying specificity may be obtained from a single fusion. However, chromosome loss may still occur during subsequent culture. The technique may also be used to select a specific isotype (see Section 4.4 for other methods) and selection may also be performed on the basis of the high DNA content of fused cells. It is a highly specialised method involving complex equipment and the selection process can readily cause cell damage. The technique may also be used for T cell hybridomas (Taniguchi and Miller, 1978; Arnold et al., 1979). It is a method which is not frequently used at the moment because of the cost and complexity of the equipment. However if chemical selection is for some reason not possible or if experience with conventional systems gives continual overgrowth despite careful early cloning (Chapter 8) and access to a FACS may be obtained, it is a powerful method well worth consideration. The appropriate equipment may be obtained from Becton-Dickinson, Sunnyvale, California.

6.3.1. Other methods of selection

If it is difficult to produce a HAT-sensitive parent myeloma line then the use of irreversible inhibitors may be considered (Chapter 3). In this technique, the two types of cell to be used are each treated with a different cell poison which will inhibit non-overlapping functions. Only the fused progeny can then survive. Wright (1978) used the irreversible inhibitors iodoacetamide and diethylpyrocarbonate and Kobayashi et al. (1982) have produced human T cell hybridomas using the irreversible inhibitors emetine and actinomycin D. Bischoff et al. (1982) have described a method for producing hybrid cells using electrofusion.

6.4. Preparation of stock solutions

6.4.1. Preparation of PEG

Weigh out 20 g PEG 1500 (Koch-Light) in a glass 20-ml universal container. Autoclave at 15 lb/sq.inch for 10 min. The PEG will now be liquid. When it is still liquid but cool enough to handle, add 30 ml RPMI. This solution is approximately 40%. Store at room temperature. The solution keeps well over periods of several months. It is usually stored in the dark.

6.4.2. Preparation of HT and HAT

Dissolve 136 mg of hypoxanthine and 39 mg thymidine in 100 ml distilled water (HT). Hypoxanthine is not very soluble but will dissolve if heated to 50–60°. Sterilise the solution by filtration. Store at −70° in small aliquots. Use 1 ml HT for each 100-ml culture medium to be made up.

Although some people actually make up complete HAT and this works well, it is usually more convenient to make up the aminopterin component (A) separately. This is for two reasons. After the control myeloma cells in a fusion have died and aminopterin is no longer necessary, hypoxanthine and thymidine (HT) should still be added for a few days to allow for medium dilution and cell adaptation. Also, it is the most labile of the three chemicals and has to be checked separately. The easiest method is therefore either to buy aminopterin already in solution (0.1 mM Flow Laboratories) or to make up and aliquot a 0.1-mM solution. This may be done by dissolving 1.8 mg aminopterin in 50 ml of 5 mM NaOH, neutralising with HCl and making up to 100 ml with distilled water. However, since 1.8 mg is not readily weighed, it is more common to dissolve 18 mg of amino-pterin in 50 ml 5 mM NaOH, neutralise with HCl and make up to 100 ml with distilled water. 10 ml of this solution are then diluted to 100 ml with distilled water to make a 0.1 mM solution. 0.4 ml of this solution is then used for every 100-ml culture medium so the solution is aliquoted in 0.4 ml amounts and stored *IN THE DARK* at $-70°$.

6.5. *Fusion frequencies and plating densities*

Fusion frequencies are discussed in more detail in Section 3.2.3. In general, these range between 1 and 100 in 10^7 lymphocytes for the rodent system and an order of magnitude lower for the human system. In a typical mouse fusion, 100 clones or more may be expected. A highly successful fusion is better handled in 96-well Costar plates at a density of 10^5 cells/well as the chances of two clones competing for the same medium are reduced and this is therefore the recommended procedure. However, a less successful fusion is better handled in 24-well Costar plates at a higher plating density. Both types of plating can also be used so that the fusion is covered for all contingencies as it is impossible to predict the success of a fusion at the start. It is easy to see mouse clones on 24-well plates as they emerge and they can be grown for longer without disturbance if they emerge as single col-onies. In addition, a fusion may be laid down in 1 ml of medium leaving room for an extra 1 ml to be added to feed the cells with minimal disturbance.

   The capacity of the 96-well plates is only 0.2 ml and it is not usual to plate cells out much below this figure for long periods of time as extensive evaporation (particularly in the outer wells) is observed. If a fusion has been seeded on 24-well Costar plates and is more successful than anticipated with multiple clones in each well, it is quite possible to aspirate the clones from a mouse fusion (but not a rat one) independently with a pasteur pipette or eppendorf tip held vertically over them. These clones may then be independently expanded and subcloned. In general, if fusions have been giving low frequencies it is useful to move to 24-well plates until the causes of the low frequency have been ascertained and overcome.

6.6. Fusion protocols for mouse experiments

There are a large number of fusion protocols in general circulation and most of them work. The major variations from the one used in our laboratory are noted below the main recommended one.

Protocol 6.1

General fusion plan for mouse hybridomas

(i) 3–6 weeks before fusion. Start immunisation schedule (Chapter 4).

(ii) 7 or more days before fusion. Make up stock solutions of HT (Section 6.4.2), A (Section 6.4.2), P/S (Section 5.2.5), freeze, and check equipment.

(iii) 7 days before fusion. The parent myeloma line should be in active logarithmic growth at the time of fusion. Grow the cells in RPMI + 10% FCS + P/S and monitor the growth rate keeping cell density in the region of 10^5 cells/ml. Do standard mycoplasma and viability checks. Plan to have in the region of 10^8 cells on fusion day at greater than 95% viability (Section 5.3.4).

(iv) 3–4 days before fusion. Boost the animal with a large dose but not so large as to induce immune paralysis (see Chapter 3).

(v) 1 day before fusion. Lay down feeder cells if they are to be used (see Section 5.5). It is not essential to lay down feeders at all and not

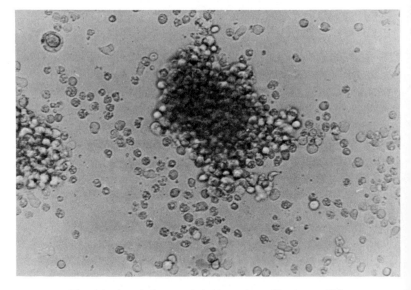

Fig. 6.2. A typical mouse hybridoma (magnification × 500).

essential the day before fusion but if they are to be used it is better to split the workload over two days. Check equipment. Sterilise instruments.

(vi) Fusion day. See Protocol 6.2.

(vii) 5–10 days after fusion. Feed the cells with HAT-containing medium.

(viii) 10–14 days after fusion. Inspect the cells for hybridoma growth (Fig. 6.2) and control cell death. Assay and proceed to subcloning (Chapter 8).

Protocol 6.2

Fusion

(i) Prepare the materials, all sterile. Thaw the FCS and HT and A. Put the RPMI and HT and A into a 37° water bath. Lay out at least two 6-cm petri dishes, three 21-G and three 25-G sterile disposable needles, two 10-ml disposable syringes, a large number (around 10) of sterile conical 20-ml universal containers, a stock of 10 each of 2-, 5- and 10-ml pipettes, a haemocytometer, two eppendorf tubes containing 0.3 ml 0.9% ammonium chloride, and the PEG solution. It is unrealistic to give exact quantities of small items as minor changes may lead to the requirement for more of any particular item. Pour some sterile RPMI into a sterile universal.

(ii) Harvest and count the myeloma cells. Check their viability. If this is below 90% postpone the fusion. It should be above 95%. Resuspend in RPMI alone if the preparation of the spleen cells is likely to occur soon thereafter. Otherwise resuspend in complete medium (10% FCS) and keep in the humidified CO_2 incubator.

(iii) Kill the animal (Appendix 1), taking a sample of blood for assay if required. *DO NOT DO THIS IN THE STERILE HOOD.* Immerse the animal in 70% ethanol, and dissect out the spleen with sterile instruments placing it in the universal containing RPMI.

(iv) Move the spleen to the sterile hood. Wash twice with serum-free RPMI and dissect off any fatty tissue. Put the spleen into a 6-cm petri dish containing 5 ml RPMI. Gently tease the spleen cells from the capsule using two 21-G needles to break up clumps. Draw the spleen cell suspension into a 10-ml pipette through a 21-G needle and pipette it out again. Repeat once with a 21-G needle and then twice with 25-G needles. Use moderate pressure only. Pipette the spleen cells directly through the 25-G needle into a universal. Centrifuge for 5 min at 500 g.

(v) Wash the spleen cell pellet twice in serum-free RPMI, resuspending the pellet with gentle tapping and centrifuging as before. Resuspend in serum-free RPMI. While the cells are centrifuging, make up complete medium (10% FCS) plus 2 × HAT if feeders have been used and 1 × HAT if there are no feeders.

(vi) Count the spleen cells. The number should be in the region of 10^8. The spleen cells are not always readily seen and the counting is improved if a 0.05-ml aliquot is pipetted into the eppendorf tube containing the 0.3 ml ammonium chloride and left for 3 min for the cells to swell and become more visible. Remember the extra dilution factor involved if you do this.

(vii) Keep a sample of both spleen cells and myeloma cells (at least 5×10^6) for use as controls. Mix the two main cell populations in serum-free medium in the ratio of 5:1 spleen:myeloma and centrifuge at 500 g for 5 min. As there are usually around 10^8 spleen cells this means that around 2×10^7 myeloma cells will be required. Pour off the supernatant gently and tap the pellet to loosen it.

(viii) Add 2 ml PEG solution evenly over a period of about half a minute shaking the cells by flicking the tube all the time. Resuspend the cells gently with a 2-ml pipette over a further half minute and then allow them to stand for 30 sec. Then add 5 ml serum-free RPMI dropwise over the next 2 min shaking the cells gently all the time. Add another 5 ml serum-free RPMI at once and leave to stand for about 3 min, then centrifuge at 500 g for 5 min.

(ix) Resuspend the cells gently in 50 ml complete medium (i.e. RPMI with 10% FCS and $2 \times$ HAT) if feeders are used or 100 ml complete medium with $1 \times$ HAT if there are no feeders. Plate out 0.5 ml (approximately 10^6 cells/well) on a 24-well Costar plate with prepared feeders and 1 ml on a Costar plate with no feeders. Plate out 0.1 ml ($1-2 \times 10^5$ cells/well) on a 96-well Costar plate with 0.1 ml feeders and 0.2 ml on a plate with no feeders. About 4–5 Costar plates of either type (Section 6.5) should be required if the spleen yielded 10^8 cells. Leave the last column of each plate for controls.

(x) Centrifuge both the control spleen cells and control myeloma cells at 500 g for 5 min and resuspend in the same medium as the fused cells. Plate out at 10^6 cells/well on 24-well Costar plates or $1-2 \times 10^5$ cells/well on 96-well Costar plates (Section 6.3) the same number of both types of cell separately preferably with a sample of both on each plate. It is useful but not essential to have controls on each plate in case a plate is lost through contamination or accident or differential growth occurs.

6.6.1. Variations on fusion protocols for mouse

It has been emphasised throughout this book that the number of variations in procedure is immense. However, some major variations in technique together with their rationales are outlined below.

Step (iv). The spleen has many cells other than B lymphocytes. If the whole spleen is put through a sieve or tea strainer then more cells will be obtained but these include many fibroblasts which can dominate the cultures. On the other hand, the rapidly dividing cells which are most likely to participate in a good fusion are mobile and a predominance of these is obtained by 'flushing out' the spleen with a combination of syringing and teasing with needles. In teasing the spleen cells apart, most of the mobile cells are obtained. This is therefore a median position and comparatively easy to perform. It may however leave clumps. Many people do not use the needle dispersion technique but a preliminary centrifugation to remove clumps. This requires very low speeds and is difficult to judge on most laboratory centrifuges. The technique of putting the cells direct from a 25-G needle into the sterile universal tube has therefore been selected.

Step (v). Some laboratories use 20% FCS where 10% is recommended here.

Step (vi). Most mouse spleens have in the region of 10^8 cells and rat spleens have about twice that number. In addition, the number of cells obtained will depend on the exact technique used to disperse the spleen cells as described in Note (iv). It is therefore quite common to dispense with this step entirely and assume that the spleen cells are in the order of 10^8 in number.

Step (vii). Controls are useful in monitoring the death of both the parent cell lines. In addition, the spleen cell control is useful in monitoring when secretion has stopped. The myeloma control is vital for the monitoring of the effectiveness of the aminopterin.

The ratio of spleen cells to myeloma cells varies in protocols from 10/1 to 2/1. In general it has declined in published protocols throughout the years. The rationales behind this relate to the extent to which the cells involved in the fusion are able to fuse and (in the case of the spleen cells) of the correct cell type. In addition, the spleen cells are often not counted. Almost any ratio works within the range described.

Step (viii). It is here that the greatest variation in technique arises. The protocol described derives from the technique of Oi and Herzenberg (1980). A common and successful variation is to centrifuge the cells for 5 min at about 200 g and then leave the pellet for a full 8 min. After gentle resuspension the cells are then pelleted again at 800 g for 5 min, the supernatant is removed and medium is added. This particular technique derives from the original work of Gefter et al. (1977) and Claflin and Williams (1978). Fazekas de St. Groth and Scheidegger (1980) have compared three totally different techniques of PEG induced fusion and found them all comparable in terms of production of fused cells. The only advice which can be given is that if good reagents are used, good results may be obtained by the recommended protocol and many others. It must be remembered that PEG is toxic to cells but also helps fusion. All the techniques described vary in their balance between these two factors.

Step (ix). For plating densities see Section 6.4.

HAT is conveniently added at this stage. Several protocols suggest that it is better to add HAT 24 h after fusion when the cells have settled. As ever, there is no detailed evidence for this and it is logical to suppose that the unfused myeloma cells will meantime have dominated the culture well. Indeed a common procedure involves the laying down of the feeders 24 h in advance with HAT and adding the fused cells to established feeders in a small volume. Excellent results may be obtained by this last method which minimises the number of manipulations required on the day of fusion.

Step (x). Controls are vital as indicated in Step (xi) itself. In particular, aminopterin is unstable and if it is not having any effect, the control myeloma cells will grow, and obviously swamp the hybridomas. Control myelomas are therefore essential. Control spleen cells are less essential but it is helpful to know whether they no longer produce a positive supernatant. It is possible to have a fusion where every supernatant is positive and this is usually due to an exceptionally effective antigen. Reference to the spleen cell control is valuable in such cases.

The general experimental approach to a fusion is probably best if the fusion itself is not regarded as critical. With a well prepared experiment only a single fusion should be necessary but with difficult antigens several fusions may be required and it is best to establish a laboratory attitude where a fusion is not a major event but only an established procedure which can be fitted in a short session of laboratory work.

6.6.2. Variations in fusion protocols for rat systems

Rat fusions are carried out in a manner similar to mouse fusions. A ratio of 2:1 spleen:myeloma cells is recommended (Galfre et al.,

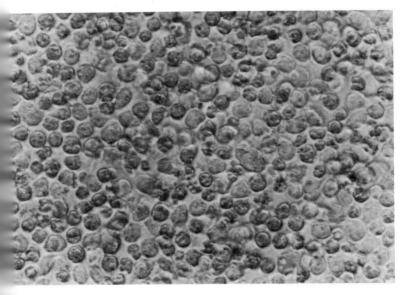

Fig. 6.3. A typical rat hybridoma (magnification × 1000). Note that well defined clones are rarely visible.

1979), and the emerging clones are diffuse and more difficult to detect (Fig. 6.3) (Chapter 8). A rat spleen usually gives 2×10^8 cells, about double that of the mouse.

6.6.3. Variations in fusion protocol for human systems

The main fusion techniques for human hybridoma production are very similar to the mouse ones. For both human–human and mouse–human fusions the ratio of myeloma cells:lymphocytes used by Cote et al. (1983) was 2:1 or 1:1. However, the LICR-LON-HMy2 line early fusions were performed at higher ratios also with success. Most human fusions incorporate 2×10^{-5} M mercaptoethanol in the complete culture medium. Selection with azaserine (0.4 µg/ml) rather than aminopterin is sometimes employed (Edwards et al., 1982) and this reduces the necessary concentration of the components of HAT required. It is claimed to give a higher yield of hybrids and is particularly useful for cells which are highly sensitive to thymidine such as T cell hybridomas (Foung et al., 1982).

Human parent myeloma lines which have been selected in azaguanine or thioguanine are usually passaged regularly with the selective drug to check for any revertant mutants.

CHAPTER 7

Transformation

7.1. Introduction

Cell transformation is potentially an extremely valuable aid to hybridoma production. At the moment it is limited to the use of viruses known to transform B lymphocytes of the appropriate species. However, advances in research into transforming genes of tumour cells are very rapid indeed and it seems to be very likely that transformation with the appropriate DNA will be possible in many systems in the near future. The greatest advantages of transformation are that it is possible to immortalise a very high percentage of antibody-producing cells so that the 'fusion frequency' is effectively increased by several orders of magnitude, and that no chemical selection is required. The main disadvantage is traditonally thought to be the loss in antibody secretion ability of transformed cells after a certain period of time. This experience is mainly based on experience with bulk cultures and under these conditions, fused cells also lose the ability to secrete, so there is as yet no firm foundation to this view. The process must nonetheless be different since fused cells can have overgrowth due to chromosome loss and transformed cells do not carry a tetraploid chromosome load. However, in general, transformed cells do tend to dedifferentiate so there may be much more complex biology in the system yet to be investigated. The most extensive research in this area has been carried out by Kozbor's group (Kozbor and Roder, 1981; Kozbor, Lagarde and Roder, 1982; Kozbor and Roder, 1983) utilising human lymphocytes making antibody to tetanus toxin and transformed with Epstein Barr virus. In principle, the same technique could be applied with murine viruses for either B cells (Moloney, 1960) or T cells (Finn et al., 1979; Ricciardi-Castagnoli et al., 1981).

7.2. Pre-selection of lymphocytes of pre-defined specificity

In general, lymphocytes are not selected for a cell fusion. This is partly for historical reasons (it was not necessary) with the early highly immunogenic antigens used in hybridoma experiments) and partly because of the numbers of cells involved. A rodent spleen has in the region of 10^8 cells of which only around 10^5 are likely to be secreting the required antibody. With a fusion frequency of around 1 in 10^6 this is likely to yield only small numbers of hybridomas. Thus, for mouse or rat fusions several animals are likely to be necessary for either in vivo or in vitro immunisation. If this is possible, then it is excellent method since an extra few hours work before the fusion can save many hours work during selection and screening as every clone which grows is of potential interest. However, it may still have lost the relevant chromosomes if the cells are fused rather than transformed.

The two types of selection procedures available are positive and negative selection. It should be emphasised that these are not totally complementary. With both fusion and transformation techniques there are probably other factors involved such as cell surface receptors for a tranorming virus or the position in the cell cycle and secretion capacity of the fused cell. These may not correlate completely with the ability to bind antigen which is the basis for selection techniques. At the moment selection procedures in general are only available for soluble antigens although Walker et al. (1977) have used a soluble preparation from sheep red blood cell membranes for this purpose

7.2.1. Pre-selection of B lymphocytes

T lymphocytes are readily removed from a human mixed lymphocyt sample by E rosetting with sheep red blood cells to leave a cell population enriched in B cells and monocytes. The most frequent application of this technique is in the transformation of human B lymphocytes with Epstein Barr virus. The majority of the human population have T lymphocytes which are cytotoxic to this virus and preliminary removal of these improves the transformation frequency. Preliminary rosetting is also used where T cells dominate the lymphocyte population to a considerable extent and removal improves the frequency of production of positive clones in a conventional fusion. There may be some situations in2.1ich helper T cells are better left in the lymphocyte population but there are no clear instances of this in hybridoma technology with the exception of in vitro immunisation techniques. The basis of the technique is that human and swine but not mouse or rabbit T cells bind to SRBCs and can consequently be separated from the rest of the peripheral blood mononuclear cells on the basis of the greater density of the erythrocytes. SRBCs alone are not an ideal reagent as preparations can be very variable and protocols usually involve SRBCs which have been pretreated with enzymes such as papain or neuraminidase or with sulphydryl reagents. The protocol given below is derived from Kaplan and Clark (1974) and is economical and reproducible.

Protocol 7.1

Rosetting of human T lymphocytes

All preparations should be undertaken under sterile conditions if the B lymphocytes are to be used for subsequent transformation or fusion.

(i) Make up Percoll (Pharmacia) at a density of 1.08 in RPMI. Weigh out 102 mg of 2-aminoethylisothiouronium bromide (AET Aldrich Chemicals) and dissolve in 10 ml distilled water. Adjust to exactly pH 9 with NaOH. Filter through a 0.2-μm filter to sterilise.

(ii) Wash 2 ml of fresh packed sheep red blood cells (SRBCs) three times with serum-free RPMI. Add 8 ml of the AET solution and incubate at 37° for 20 min with occasional shaking. Add RPMI and centrifuge at 500 g for 5 min. Wash the cells at least 5 times in RPMI, and resuspend in RPMI at a concentration of 10%. This preparation is stable for up to 5 days.

(iii) Dilute the stored AET-treated SRBCs to 2%. Wash the lymphocytes to be separated in serum-free RPMI and then, in order, add equal volumes of the 2% AE teated SRBCs, RPMI and FCS. The cells tend to clump with FCS which is added last. Centrifuge at 200 g for 10 min. Do not remove the supernatant but incubate the tube for 90 min in an ice bath.

(iv) Resuspend by gently rocking the tube. Count the rosettes on the haemocytometer. About 60% of the PBLs should have formed rosettes.

(v) Layer the cells very gently onto an equal volume of Percoll (Pharmacia) and centrifuge at 500 g for 15 min. The rosetted T lymphocytes should pellet to the bottom of the tube and the B lymphocytes should remain at the interface. If the SRBCs fail to pellet this is more likely to be because the tube has been spun too fast rather than too slow as Percoll forms very steep gradients. Harvest the B lymphocytes and wash with RPMI twice.

(vi) If the T lymphocytes in the pellet are required, the SRBCs are readily lysed with 5-sec exposure to distilled water followed by immediate addition of medium.

7.2.2. Positive selection (Fig. 7.1)

Positive selection of antigen-specific lymphocytes is readily performed with soluble antigens. These are attached to sheep red blood cells and the mixture is centrifuged in Percoll. The relevant lymphocytes are conveniently located in the resulting pellet. If the SRBCs are 'tanned', although they will not lyse they will not disturb transformation. Nevertheless, they will almost certainly disturb fusion. If they are coated but not tanned, then the SRBCs are readily lysed. However, the ability to bind antigen does not always correlate with the ability of the cells to make antibodies specific for the antigen (Nossal

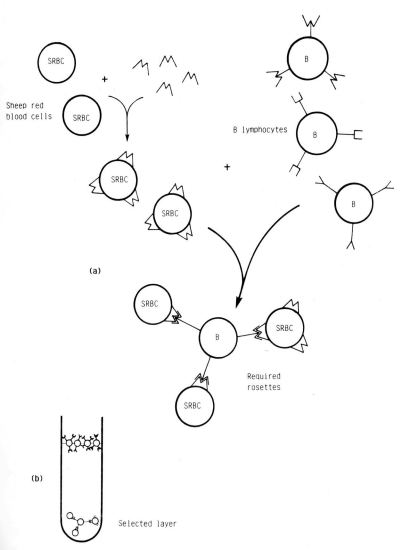

Fig. 7.1. Positive selection. The antigen is bound to sheep red blood cells and the relevant lymphocytes are selected by rosetting on Ficoll. (a) Theory; (b) practice.

and Pike, 1976; Kozbor and Roder, 1981). Positive selection may also be performed by use of the fluorescent activated cell sorter (Section 6.3) and by other varieties of solid and liquid phase techniques (reviewed by Basch et al., is 1983). Positive selection may of course be applied after as well as before fusion (Chapter 8).

Protocol 7.2

Positive selection

(i) Make up Percoll in RPMI at a density of 1.08. Make a 1% (w/v) solution of hydrated chromic chloride in 0.15 M sodium chloride at pH 5. Some laboratories prefer to 'age' this solution for 2–3 weeks, maintaining the pH at 5.

(ii) Prepare a 1 mg/ml solution of the soluble protein antigen.

(iii) If human blood is the source of the lymphocytes to be selected, prepare the B lymphocytes by rosetting the T lymphocytes (Protocol 7.3) from 50–100 ml blood. 10 ml blood should yield in excess of 10^7 lymphocytes of which about 20% are B lymphocytes. A mouse spleen should yield 10^8 cells of which less than 50% are B lymphocytes.

(iv) Use a preparation of sheep red blood cells not more than two weeks old. Wash by centrifugation at 500 g in 0.15 M NaCl at least three times and more if the supernatant remains red. Take 0.5 ml packed cell volume and dilute to 4.5 ml in 0.15 M saline.

(v) Add 0.5 ml of the antigen solution.

(vi) Dilute the chromic chloride solution 1 in 100 with 0.15 M saline and add 5 ml of this dropwise to the antigen–erythrocyte solution with constant mixing. Continue to mix for a period of 15 min. Then add 10 ml phosphate-buffered saline, mix and centrifuge at 500 g for 5 min. Wash the pellet twice with phosphate-buffered saline.

(vii) The coated SRBCs may then be used to isolate antigen binding B cells. The procedure is identical with that in Protocol 7.1, steps (iii) to (vi). The antigen-specific B cells will be in the SRBC pellet while the rest will be in the interface.

7.2.3. *Negative selection* (Fig. 7.2)

This procedure was developed by Walker et al. (1977). It is based on the premise that B lymphocytes exposed to saturing concentrations of antigen 'cap' i.e. lose their surface immunoglobulin. B cells which have not done this will react with SRBCs conjugated to the Fab fraction of the appropriate anti-immunoglobulin. These cells may then be removed by gradient centrifugation leaving behind a B cell population enriched for the appropriate specificity. In cases where the subsequent response is enhanced by macrophages or T cells this technique has an obvious advantage in that these cells also remain behind. However, if the enriched B cell population is to be subsequently transformed as in the case of EB virus with human cells, the T lymphocytes are better removed as they may be cytotoxic to the virus.

Protocol 7.3

Negative selection

(i) Using protocol 7.2., prepare SBCs coated with the $F(ab)_2$ fraction of anti-human IgG (Cappel Laboratories). The $F(ab)_2$ fragment may also be made by digesting 50 mg of IgG with 1 mg pepsin in 0.1 M Na acetate pH 5 with subsequent recovery of the $F(ab)_2$ fragment as the first peak on a Sephadex G200 column (Johnstone and Thorpe, 1982). The use of the whole immunoglobulin molecule for coupling is not recommended as non-specific binding may be obtained due to Fc receptors on non-specific PBLs.

(ii) Incubate the B lymphocytes or PBLs with antigen in RPMI for 1 h. The antigen should be at saturating concentration i.e. $100 \, \mu g/10^7$ cells/ml for a soluble protein antigen. Wash the cells twice in RPMI by centrifugation and resuspend in complete medium. Incubate for at least 3 h.

(iii) Using the $F(ab)_2$-coated SRBCs, proceed as in Protocol 7.1 steps (iii) to (vi). The lymphocytes of the chosen antigen specificity will be obtained from the interface layer.

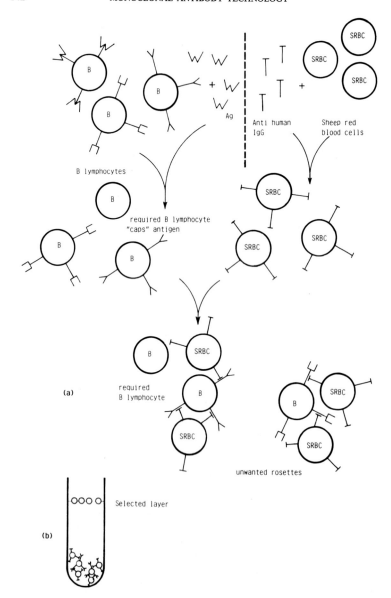

7.3. Pre-selection of T lymphocytes

Either pre-selection or enrichment of T lymphocytes before fusion is frequently employed. This is particularly relevant where selection or assay procedures after fusion relate to cell-surface antigens as a B–T fusion may be confused with T–T fusion (Taussig et al., 1980). Enrichment is usually by the use of nylon fibre which binds B but not T cells (Greaves and Brown, 1974) or by the use of plates coated with anti-immunoglobulin of the appropriate species. T cells purified in this way are often further cloned in the presence of growth factors before fusion is attempted (Beezley and Ruddle, 1982; Haas and Von Boehmer, 1982).

7.4. Transformation

The only system currently extensively utilised for transformation is the Epstein Barr virus (EB) system discussed in Section 3.6.4. This is totally specific for human B lymphocytes and has been known for many years. No published work on any other system is yet available so the protocol for this system is given. In general, it is similar to the systems used for fusion except that pre-selected cells are generally used and cloning is applied from the start of the experiment. The protocol is given without pre-selection which is strongly advised. With the EB system, it is necessary to remove cytotoxic T lymphocytes since these are present in most donors. If transforming genes or rare transforming viruses are used this may be less important. The use of AET-treated SRBCs for the removal of T lymphocytes (Kaplan et al., 1974) is recommended as it results in enhanced T cell binding. The

Fig. 7.2. Negative selection. The antigen is incubated with the lymphocytes which then 'cap' (i.e. internalise the surface antibody). Sheep red blood cells coated with antibody to human IgG are then incubated with the lymphocytes. Only the non-specific lymphocytes rosette as the rest have temporarily internalised their Ig. The specific ones can then be selected at the interface of a Percoll gradient. (a) Theory; (b) practice.

technique could also be used to isolate the relevant T lymphocytes. Feeder cells are generally during transformation but are not strictly necessary. However they are necessary for cloning.

Protocol 7.4.

The Epstein Barr transformation system. Overall plan

(i) Obtain B95-8 cells (Chapter 3). Check for mycoplasma. Grow in RPMI + 10% FCS + P/S (see Chapter 3). The supernatant of this cell line (which is of marmoset origin) secretes EB virus. The cell line is propagated in 25-cm^2 flasks, the supernatant is filtered through 0.45-μm filters and stored in 1-ml aliquots in an eppendorf tube inside a universal at −70 °C. Several aliquots of virus containing supernatant should be available at any time.

(ii) Find a suitable human donor, negative for EB virus antibodies, for the supply of feeder cells. It is not clear how important this is but most laboratories report substantially better growth on feeder cells from an EBV negative source. Only about 1 in 10 of the human population is EB negative (see Chapter 5 for methods). The donor must be someone willing and readily available.

If it is not possible to find a donor, then a variety of other feeder systems (see Chapter 5) may be investigated. Cells will grow on the peripheral blood lymphocytes (PBLs) of an EB positive donor but very much less vigorously. It is likely that a T cell response is involved and human B lymphocytes may also prove to be suitable feeders whoever the donor.

(iii) Take 20–50 ml blood from the human donor of the appropriate antibody specificity. The specific donor does not need to be EB negative. Frequently, the finding of the appropriate donor involves extensive clinical liaison and frequently the appropriate cells are not available on the chosen fusion day (for example the day in which a tumour is removed). For fusion this may be a drawback but for transformation the lymphocytes may be frozen in the same way as tissue-culture (10% DMSO, 20% FCS). In general, however, fresh cells yield better results. Cells from patients at high titre are not always the best, since what is required is *proliferating* cells of the appropriate specificity.

(iv) 1 day before transformation prepare AET-treated SRBCs (Protocol 7.1). Prepare feeder feeder cell suspension. Take 20 ml of PBLs from the EB negative donor, rosette out the T cells (Protocol 7.1) and irradiate the feeders at 2000 R. (Mouse macrophages at 10^4 cells/well are also reported to good feeders). Lay down feeders at 5×10^4 cells/well in flat bottomed 96-well Costar plates or 10^4 cells/well in round bottomed 96-well Costar plates.

(v) Transformation day. With fresh blood from appropriate human donor, prepare the PBLs and then the B cells by rosetting out the T cells on SRBCs (see Protocol 7.1). Pre-select (Protocols 7.2 and 7.3) and transform. With frozen PBLs, pre-select, and then transform (see Protocol 7.5).

(vi) Ignore the cells for at least 10 days unless you suspect contami-

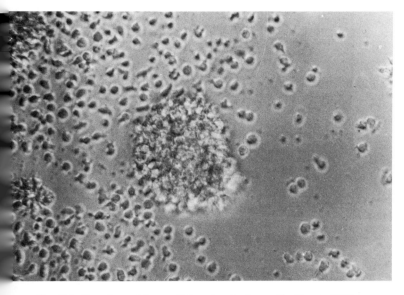

Fig. 7.3. Transformed human B lymphocytes (magnification × 1000).

nation (see Chapter 5). If the cells are transformed they will change shape from round to oblong (or panhandle) shape (Fig. 7.3), and will obviously be growing. After 2-3 weeks, they should be subcloned on the same feeder cells preferably from the same donor.

(vii) Subclone as described in Chapter 8.

Protocol 7.5

Transformation of cells with EB virus

(i) Take at least 20 ml (for pre-selection at least 200 ml) of blood from the appropriate donor. Remove T lymphocytes (Protocol 7.1). This should leave around 8×10^6 cells from 20 ml blood. The cells may be frozen in liquid nitrogen at this stage. Pre-select according to Protocols 7.2 or 7.3. Resuspend the B lymphocytes (which may have monocytes among them) in the B95-8 cell supernatant (see Protocol 7.4(i)) at a concentration of around 10^7 cells/ml. Incubate at 37° for 1 h. Centrifuge the cells at 500 g for 5 min and wash in RPMI.

(ii) Resuspend the cells in RPMI + 10% FCS + P/S (complete medium) at 10^6 cells/ml. Then, make up doubling dilutions in complete medium over a 6-fold range i.e. 0.5×10^6 cells, 2.5×10^6 cells/ml, etc. This is most conveniently performed by having for each plate 2 ml at the highest concentration. The cells are plated out in 0.1-ml aliquots into rows B2 to B11, the outer wells being filled with distilled water. The remaining 1 ml is then diluted to 2 ml with medium and used to aliquot 0.1-ml samples into rows C2 to C11 and so on.

Note. EB virus is only a Category C pathogen and can be handled with routine microbiological precautions. However, it should be noted that particularly when the B95-8 cell supernatant is being handled there is a high titre present. It is probably wise to wear disposable gloves at least at this stage and to use autoclavable plasticware which is placed in a bag in the hood. This is also good practice with relatively untested donors as all human blood samples have to be treated as potential sources of hepatitis.

7.5. *Transformation followed by fusion*

Most human antibody secreting cells made immortal by transformation have been made from donors with a high natural level of antibody such as those to blood group antigens or by extensive immunisation with soluble proteins such as tetanus toxin. Even in these cases, there is no guarantee of any stability in the antibody secretion of these transformants. For this reason, 'back fusion' with either mouse or human myelomas is an obvious precautionary measure to take to ensure that the resulting hybridoma continues to make the appropriate antibody. There is no clear rationale behind this. Kozbor and Roder (1981) showed that clones of transformed human B lymphocytes which did not secrete tetanus toxin specific antibody, grew no faster than those which did. However, it is quite possible that within any particular culture well, overgrowth by non-antibody secreting cells occurs. This does not mean that the non-secretors grow fast or that they are true non-secretors but rather than that their antibody is irrelevant to the antigen in question and that unfortunately they grow faster than the clones secreting the required relevant antibody. Alternatively, it may be that the cells which are largely IgM secretors, reach a stage at which they are unable to go through the isotype switch without the appropriate stimulus and consequently cease to secrete. Transformed cells fuse exceptionally well as they are growing and replicating fast. It is better for the moment to attempt to preserve the secretion of EB transformed cell lines by back fusion with a line known to have high secretion properties. Ideally, this should be a plasmocytoma line and these are readily available in the murine system. The only well characterised available human plasmocytoma line is the SKO-007 and Cote et al. (1983) have shown that this is not superior to mouse lines in the production of normal human monoclonal antibodies. Indeed, it seems doubtful if any human plasmocytoma line is preferable to a human lymphoblastoid cell line. Back fusion with mouse is supposed to lead to unstable clones also so that the possessor of a good human transformed line which he feels may be unstable is faced with the possibillity of fusing this with a mouse line which may also be unstable. Encouragement may be obtained from the work of Cote et al. (1983) who find mouse – human hybridomas easier to handle and more stable (and safer) than human ones. It should also be remembered that back fusions may be better performed with hybridomas specific for the human lambda light chain. This is coded by chromosome 22 which is preferentially retained in human–mouse myeloma fusions (though not human–mouse fibroblast fusions) (Croce et al., 1980).

7.5.1. Mouse human fusions of transformed human cells

This procedure can readily be accomplished by using a mouse myeloma line which is HAT-sensitive and a transformed human line secreting antibody of the required specificity. The human cells are killed by ouabain at relatively low doses (10^{-7} M) and the mouse cells, which are resistant to ouabain at doses of 10^{-5} M are killed by the aminopterin so that only the hybrids survive. As noted above, it is better to select a human line which secretes lambda light chains for this purpose. Ouabain resistance is usually of intermediate strength in the hybrids.

Protocol 7.6

Back fusion with mouse cells

(i) Make up a stock solution of 10^{-3} M ouabain. This will be used at a dilution of 1 in 100. Test for growth in complete medium (10% FCS + P/S) of both mouse myeloma parent and transformed human parent. At 10^{-5} M ouabain, the former should grow well and the latter should die rapidly.

(ii) Take the highest dilution on the plate of transformed cells which gives positive results with the antigen. Transfer to a 2-ml well of a 24-well Costar plate and grow until there are between 10^6 and 10^7 cells/well.

(iii) Subclone at least 5×96-well plates at 10 transformed cells/well or lower on irradiated human feeder cells (10^4 cells/well in round-bottomed plates, 5×10^4 cells/well on flat-bottomed plates).

(iv) Grow a further 10^5 cells in a 2-ml well of a 24-well Costar plate. There are effectively an insurance against a failed fusion but may also be a source of antibody for several months of longer.

(v) Use the remainder of the cells for a fusion with the mouse myeloma cells. The Protocol should be identical to that described in Protocol 6.2 step (vii) onwards except that the fusion ratio should be 1:1 human:mouse and ouabain at 10^{-5} M should be incorporated into the medium. Control cells of both human and mouse origin are particularly important. If feeder cells are used they should be from a mouse source. Plating out should be on 96-well plates at a cell density of 10^5 downwards as in Protocol 7.5.

(vi) Assay, expand and clone as for a conventional mouse fusion.

(vii) Repeat the procedure with any positive clones obtained from step (ii).

Protocol 7.5 is designed to rescue cells before they cease to secrete. If the cells have been pre-selected (Protocol 7.2) then this should be a suitable procedure. However in situations where it is not possible to select (i.e. tumour cell antigens) it must be remembered that the proportion of cells secreting antibody of the required specificity will be small. It is common in these situations to have a positive well at a dilution of 10^4 and a negative at the wells of higher dilution, implying that there is only a single antibody secreting cell type among 10^4 others in that well. Thus the back fusion is better performed after cloning and this is why cloning is also recommended in Protocol 7.5 step (ii). If positive clones are obtained at this stage and the cloning density was 10 cells/well or lower, the chances of obtaining a good hybridoma by back fusion are greatly increased. Cloning procedures and times for this system are given in Chapter 8. It must be emplasised that with all cloning but especially with the human system there will be very many negative clones and many plates must be assayed to detect the required positive one.

7.5.2. Human–human fusions of transformed human cells

In order to select only the hybrid cells in this system, it is necessary to fuse with a human parent line which has the appropriate drug markers. While most human cells are sensitive to ouabain, it is possible to render them relatively insensitive by a procedure of mutagenesis and growth in gradually increasing concentrations of ouabain. This has been performed by Kozbor et al. (1982) and the resulting KR-4 cell line is available if the appropriate guarantees are signed. Alternatively, it is possible ro adapt other human HAT-sensitive hybridomas to ouabain resistance. It should, however, be noted that the use of gradually increasing concentrations may lead to gene amplification and this is a relatively unstable system. It is also wise to keep thioguanine in the selection medium since mutagenesis may encourage back selection. Fusion should be as in Protocol 7.6. Mouse or human feeders may be used. In this situation there is no known need to select for lambda chain secretors.

CHAPTER 8

Selection and cloning

8.1. Early feeding and assay of fusions

Laboratory protocols vary widely in their recommendations about feeding. The following principles should be noted:

(i) Aminopterin inhibits many normal cell functions and should be removed from the feeding medium as soon as possible. The time to do this can best be judged by monitoring the myeloma control wells. In the rodent system, these are frequently dead within 10–14 days and it may never be necessary to feed a fusion with medium containing aminopterin at all. In addition, feeding at early stages is better performed (to avoid disturbance of emerging clones) if fresh medium is added without total removal of old medium and in consequence residual aminopterin will probably remain, despite its instability. If the control cells are dead, it is therefore recommended that the feeding medium should not contain aminopterin. Conversely, aminopterin is one of the least stable components of the feeding medium and sometimes it is clear from the inspection of the myeloma cells at 4 days after fusion that it has not been effective. Medium with fresh aminopterin may be added at this stage. It is vital to monitor the control wells at all times.

(ii) One single surviving myeloma cell in any culture well is likely to outgrow the hybridomas. With delicate fusions, such as human ones, this is an important factor and human hybridomas are usually maintained in aminopterin or azaserine containing medium for several weeks after fusion.

(iii) After the aminopterin is removed, hypoxanthine and thymidine should still be supplied for at least a week. Not only may residual aminopterin remain in the medium, but the emerging cells may need time to adapt to the main pathways of purine and pyrimidine biosynthesis.

(iv) Fast growing clones are indicated by the change in pH (i.e. yellow medium). These should be fed.

(v) Every tissue-culture operation increases the risk of contamination and may disturb the growing clones. Thus feeding should be as infrequent as possible.

(vi) All clones should be assayed and subcloned as early as possible.

(vii) Change of medium designed to feed the cells also removes the antibody they produce. At the same time, the amount of antibody produced in the early stages of clonal growth may be too small to be detected by the assay system.

It is quite obvious that most of these criteria cannot be satisfied by the same feeding schedule as they are frequently in conflict. Published protocols vary widely in their advice on the care of clones at this stage presumably because the laboratories involved have produced hybridomas which grow at varying rates and also because differential weight is put on some of the main principles outlined. Fazekas de St. Groth and Scheidegger (1980) noted some of these wide variations in feeding schedules and attempted to make a comparison. While their comparison has limited statistical significance and could be considered outdated by the fast development of hybridoma technology their conclusions were that hybridomas given the least attention (i.e. no feeding until 7–10 days) performed best. Other variation relates to how great a proportion (if any) of the medium is removed and replaced during feeding and this in turn may vary with the type of feeder cell, the size of Costar plate, the percentage of FCS used in the original fusion, and as has been mentioned frequently, the likelihood of contamination being introduced by the operator or cell-handling conditions. A 7-day schedule is recommended in this book for rodent fusions and it undoubtedly works. There is no clear difference in published schedules for human cells except that they may take longer to develop into visible clones (Cote et al., 1983) and even in 1983 some protocols (Olsson et al.) recommend 3-day feeding rather than 7-day feeding which is used by most others (Edwards et al., 1982; Cote et al., 1983). Since all these seem to produce hybridomas it is difficult to recommend a consensus schedule. The home laboratory, however, operates on an infrequent feeding schedule and this may bias the protocols somewhat.

Protocol 8.1 tries to incorporate some of the highly conflicting requirements listed together with the published experience. It should not be rigidly adhered to but rather adapted according to the rate of hybridoma growth and considerations (i) to (vii).

Protocol 8.1

Post fusion care of hybridomas

(i) Inspect the cells after 4–5 days. There should be massive cell death and the Costar plate should be a scene of devastation. However, it may be possible to discern some live cells in the test wells and none in the control wells. Do not feed unless there is obvious cell growth which is unlikely. If the control myelomas look healthy, however, feed with complete medium (10% FCS) + HAT using fresh aminopterin.

(ii) After 7–10 days the cells should be fed. If 24-well Costar plates have been used then it is possible to add an additional 1 ml medium if the feeder and fusion protocols in Chapters 5 and 6 have been used. If, however, a 96-well plate has been used then each well will already contain the optimal 0.2 ml of medium and half the medium (0.1 ml) must be removed before feeding. Feeding should be with complete medium (10% FCS) + HT. If the control cells are not completely dead or if there is any doubt at all about them, aminopterin should also be added. If the fusion is human, then aminopterin should be retained in the feeding medium for at least 4–6 weeks.

(iii) Between 8 and 14 days (longer for human fusions) visible clones may appear. In a mouse fusion they are readily identified. In a rat fusion they are much harder to detect. Human fusions vary with the cell line used but it is advisable to check how for possible transformed cells if the parent lymphocyte donor was Epstein Barr positive (see Protocol 7.3). When the clones are approximately 1 mm in diameter the medium in the well can be assayed for antibody content. Remove 1 ml (24-well plates) or 0.1 ml (96-well plates) for assay and replace with complete medium (10% FCS) + HT. If no clones are visible by 14 days the medium should be changed anyway so 1 ml (24-well plates) or 0.1 ml (96-well plates) should be removed, assayed and replaced with fresh medium. It is important to assay the spleen cell controls also at this time as they will give an indication of the background antibody level due to antibody secretion from unfused spleen cells.

If a fusion shows no obvious growth after 14 days it is not lost but may just be slow. It should be fed and assayed every 7–10 days by changing half the medium and maintained for up to 6 weeks (7 for human). If it shows no growth by that time, it probably never will.

8.2. Failure of fusions

Fusions may fail for obvious reasons such as contamination or equipment failure. Poor aminopterin will lead to failure but this is readily detected by growth in the myeloma control wells. In some cases however, protocols are faithfully adhered to, the control cells die, and no hybridoma is obtained. Such failures divide naturally into two groups.

8.2.1. Failure where clonal growth is good

If a fusion showed good growth but gave no positive wells then both the primary immunogen and the assay used for antibody detection should be examined closely. It may be that both worked well to yield and detect antibody in polyclonal sera but not monoclonal antibodies.

The differences in assay likely to be encountered are discussed in Chapter 2 but the most likely problems are:

(i) The antigen required is a very minor component of the main immunogen and the fusion has been dominated by stronger antigens. This means that the antigen must be further purified from the original immunogen for the next attempt or that some new selection procedure must be adopted. If the titre of the original animal was high this is unlikely. If it was below 1 in 1000 this is a possible source of difficulty.

(ii) The assay (Chapter 2) was unsuitable for monoclonal antibodies. If the animal itself gave a high titre then the assay system should be dissected in detail. For example an assay system dependent on the location of two dissimilar epitopes in close proximity is unsuitable. An over-specific second antibody may also cause problems. In theory any anti-IgG suitably labelled may act as a second antibody but if the anti-IgG is raised to a specific mouse immunoglobulin type, then it relies on determinants on the constant region of the light (usually kappa in mouse) chain for detection of other types. These may be inaccessible or low in number. Commercial second antibodies vary widely in quality as well as specificity and this should be examined closely.

8.2.2. Failure with no clonal growth

Most people react wrongly to this type of failure. They tend to make minor changes in medium or PEG or fusion technique often on casual advice and hope that this will provide the magic ingredient. It has already been emphasised (Chapter 6) that almost any cells will fuse and with almost any brand of PEG dissolved in anything from distilled water to complex media and that most additives to the medium are unnecessary for clonal growth. However, it is a sensible precaution to check all calculations – for example an error of one order of magnitude in thymidine concentration in either direction will almost certainly result in a failed fusion.

The most likely problem lies in the myeloma cell line e.g. a mycoplasma contamination (see Chapter 5 for detection and cure), or poor myeloma growth at the time of fusion. Other problems may relate to pyogens or other toxic materials in the reagents. An elementary student given the correct materials can perform a fusion with reasonable growth and the quickest and most effective way of coping with this type of failure is to change every reagent, especially the myeloma cells, substituting either new ones or reagents from a group whose fusions have been successful in the last month. It is quite common for a laboratory to have success for several months and then failure for as long a period so the immediate record of a laboratory is more important than the long-term one. Even within a research group one individual may fail where others succeed and this is a reason for encouraging separate reagents and cell lines.

8.2.3. How to cope with a fusion which is too successful

If the fusion was in 24-well Costar plates then it is obvious that positive clones should be aspirated as soon as possible and either subcloned or expanded in 24-well plates for subcloning as soon as possible. Fusions which are 100% antigen positive can also occur in 96-well plates though more rarely and the first step is probably to check whether the number of cells laid down was of the correct order of magnitude. The control spleen cell wells should also be monitored to ascertain that they are negative.

Subcloning of each required clone should take at least 4 plates (see Section 8.3). Thus a highly successful fusion cannot be handled readily since there is not usually operator time or incubator space for more than about 100 plates.

If the antibody required is high affinity, then the amount of immunoglobulin secreted in relation to the size of the response should be tested i.e. if a good response is given by a small amount of antibody then the antibody is more likely to be of high affinity (see Chapters 2 and 10 for caveats). The best approach is probably to select around 10 good producers for subcloning and freeze the rest. A procedure for freezing whole-tissue-culture plates has been published (Wells and Price, 1983) though this procedure only relates to subcloned cells, and many nitrogen storage containers cannot accommodate large numbers of plates. There is no option at this point but to propagate the chosen clones and freeze the others. In the rat system this is reported to be a highly successful strategy because of the lower rate of loss of antibody secretion (Chapter 3). If one fusion was too successful, the next one may also be and clones directed at different determinants may be selected in a second fusion (Chapter 10).

8.3. Cloning of hybridomas

8.3.1. Introduction

Most people lose their hybridomas between the stages of detecting positive supernatants and cloning. The reasons are unknown, but in contrast to most other aspects of hybridomas technology, opinion on the importance of cloning early is unanimous. The principles behind this are:

(i) Fused cells carry a tetraploid number of chromosomes. They therefore have to put more energy into DNA replication. A cell which loses unnecessary chromosomes might be thought able to replicate its DNA and divide faster and be able to outgrow its neighbours. Among the chromosomes which it loses may be the ones coding for the antibody required. While this hypothesis may be correct, it has little foundation in cell-culture technology or in comparison with other systems. For example, human HeLa cells carry a massive chromosome overload but dominate almost any other human cell culture. Furthermore, transformed lymphocytes which have similar chromosome complements also show loss of secretion in uncloned cultures.

(ii) In a plasma lymphocyte as much as half of the protein synthesising apparatus may be occupied with the synthesis of immunoglobulin. Thus fused cells making antibody divert so much energy into this process that they inevitably have less energy left for division and multiplication. Consequently cells not secreting the appropriate antibody are overgrown. This may well be true but there is little evidence to prove it. Frequently overgrowth is by cells making large amounts of antibody but not of the desired specificity.

There is therefore no single logical explanation for the fact that early cloning is essential but experience undoubtedly shows this to be the case. General tissue-culture experience does, however, show that it is almost impossible for two cell lines to co-exist in the same culture medium without overgrowth by one or the other and it is best just to assume that any cell line needs to grow alone.

8.3.2. Cloning by limiting dilution

The theoretical approach to cloning by limiting dilution is based on the Poisson distribution

$$a = e^{-b}$$

a is the fraction of wells with no growth, b is the number of clones/well, e has the customary mathematical notation.

Thus, as described by Goding (1980) if $b = 1$ then $a = 0.37$ i.e. if 37% of the wells show no growth then the probability is that those which show growth have true monoclonal hybridomas in them. Cloning efficiency, correctly interpreted, is the ratio of theoretical potential cell growth to that experienced practically, expressed as a percentage.

The practical approach is more pragmatic. The potential hybridoma must not be lost. Freshly cloned cells are delicate and need company. Most mouse hybridomas tend to clump so one is likely to pipette them in groups whatever the intention. If the entire population of a positive well is seeded at 0.3 cells/well then however good the feeders, the hybridoma may be lost. In principle this should not happen if enough clones are made and this involves the use of several tissue-culture plates at each seeding density for all positive wells from the initial fusion. This in turn involves a large number of assays (although it is only necessary to assay wells with positive growth). There is little doubt that the best approach to cloning would be to seed large numbers of cells on several plates of good feeders at 0.3

cells/well or lower. However, it is possible to produce cloned hybridomas under much less stringent conditions and if the tissue-culture system for the subcloning has minor defects a great deal of effort may be expended to no effect. If cloning is undertaken at higher cell concentrations it is not really correct cloning and the hybridoma should be recloned several more times (this should be done in any case). The recommended cloning procedure is therefore to seed the hybridomas at 3, 1 and 0.3 cells/well. Indeed a batch at 10 cells/well is best used for the first cloning to test the system, although it must be emphasised that these cells are in no way cloned (the phrase 'low density cloning' is sometimes used in these cases and should not be confused with limiting dilution cloning). At least two and preferably more plates of feeders should be used for each cell density i.e. 0.3, 3, 10 cells/well; this should not lead to an immense assay load at the end of the cloning as growth will occur in comparatively few wells, especially at the lower cell density. By using the higher cell density the chances of hybridoma survival are maximised. If the hybridoma exhibits robust growth then only the plates at lower cell density need be assayed and selected. While the technical proof of monoclonality is discussed in Chapter 10, the operational proof is always evident early on at the cell culture level as a good hybridoma grows, clones well, and still secretes after a year in culture.

Limiting dilution is the choice of cloning for most people. It can be argued that because of cell clumping it is never definitive but the final proof can easily be demonstrated in the antibody produced (Chapter 10). With many human fusions, it seems to be the practice not to clone at all (Sikora et al., 1982; Warrenius et al., 1983). It remains to be seen if such hybridomas will survive. For the moment this is not recommended however dramatic the short-term gains may appear to be. It is, however, a wise precaution to maintain the parent well in growth while subcloning. It will usually stop secreting after some time but can be used again if the first subcloning fails although the number of positive subclones will be much reduced.

Protocol 8.2

Cloning by limiting dilution

(i) Select positive wells by assay (see Chapter 2 and Protocol 8.1).

(ii) Lay down the feeder cell of choice (see Chapter 5) in 96-well Costar plates. Use *at least* 6 plates for high dilution cloning which is strongly recommended (Section 8.3.2). Fewer plates may be used if cloning is to be at above 1 cell/well. Feeders may be laid down the day before cloning or on the same day.

(iii) Lay out complete medium ($+10\%$ FCS + P/S), the cell-counting chamber, automatic pipettes delivering 0.1–0.2 ml and a large supply of sterile tips for these (20–50).

(iv) Aspirate and count the cells from the positive wells. A very small number (10^3) should be required for cloning. Return the others together to a well of a 24-well Costar plate, marking it carefully.

(v) Suspend in cells to be cloned at 30 cells/ml in complete medium and plate out in 0.1-ml aliquots into two 96-well plates of feeders. Dilute the remaining cells to 10 cells/ml and repeat with a further two plates of feeders. Dilute the remainder again to 3 cells/ml and repeat. Incubate for 2–3 weeks until visible clones appear. Assay, select and reclone.

(vi) Continue to expand the uncloned parent culture in firstly a 24-well Costar plate and then a 25-cm^2 flask. Feeders should not be necessary. Freeze aliquots of $1-5 \times 10^6$ cells as early as possible as described in Section 5.3.3. Assay fairly frequently to monitor antibody secretion which in the mouse system is likely to decline rapidly.

8.3.3. Cloning in soft agar

Soft-agar cloning is now less frequently used than limiting-dilution cloning. In theory, it is a more certain method of ascertaining that the final clone is truly monoclonal as limiting dilution always carries the risk of two cells rather than one having been put into a single well. However it is also argued that the mobility of hybridoma cells is such that an apparently single clone in soft agar may originate from more than one cell although at the appropriate dilution this is highly unlikely. In practice the reason that soft agar has become less popular probably relates to the different technique required as limiting-dilution procedures are very similar to those involved in the original fusion. In addition, more early hybridoma experiments involved haemolytic assay techniques which could be used directly on the agar (Kohler and Milstein, 1975). Most other assays necessitate the picking off and subsequent growth of emergent clones in liquid medium and this is more labour intensive.

Soft agar presents technical difficulties in that it is necessary to have molten agar for the suspension of the cells and the cells are obviously vulnerable to damage at temperatures above 37°. In addition, batches of agar are highly variable and some may be toxic. Civin and Banquerigo (1983) have described cloning in tubes of low temperature gelation agar which circumvents both of these problems and may prove more suitable than the conventional agar cloning described.

In soft agar cloning the cells are grown in an upper layer of 0.25–0.3 % agar over a lower layer of 0.5 % agar. Either layer can contain feeder cells and although this is not necessary, it is recommended in Protocol 8.3. Macrophages are the best feeders in this system.

Protocol 8.3

Cloning in soft agar

(i) Prepare a 1 % solution of Bacto agar (Difco) in distilled water. Autoclave, cool to 50° and mix with an equal volume of 2 × RPMI. This preparation can be stored in 100-ml aliquots and FCS (10 %) and P/S added shortly before use.

(ii) Prepare feeder cells (Chapter 5). Make up spleen feeders at 10^8 cells/ml or macrophage feeders at 4×10^6 cells/ml (in both the cases this should be the number of cells obtained from a single mouse/ml).

(iii) Melt 100 ml stock agar and medium solution, add the FCS and P/S and cool. To 50 ml of this, add the feeder cells when the temperature is below 40°. Plate immediately in 5-ml aliquots into

10×6 cm petri dishes. Allow the agar to gel.

(iv) Count the hybridoma cells from a positive well and make 2×1-ml aliquots in a 24-well Costar plate at dilutions of 20, 50, 100, 200 and 250 cells/well if there are enough cells. Otherwise make only single 1-ml aliquots at each dilution. As in Protocol 8.2 keep some of the parent hybridoma for expansion and freezing.

(v) Add 0.5 ml of the agar in complete medium at a temperature of 40° or lower to each well and transfer immediately to the prepared petri dishes. Incubate at 37° in a well humidified incubator inspecting the dishes for clonal growth every second or third day.

(vi) Aspirate visible clones with a sterile pasteur pipette or eppendorf tip and transfer to a 24-well costar plate containing 1 ml complete medium. Check for growth and antibody production after a few days.

8.3.4. Cloning by the Fluorescence Activated Cell Sorter

Both B and T cell hybridomas may be selected for cell surface antigens or DNA content after cell fusion. The techniques are discussed in more detail in Section 6.3.

8.3.5. Cloning of human cells. Additional considerations

Human cells are usually cloned by limiting dilution and protocols such as Protocol 3.2 may be used. The difference lies in the feeder cells and this is discussed in Sections 5.5.5 and 5.5.6. Human cells are much harder to clone and plates at higher cell density such as 10 cells/well are usually included in the procedure as a precautionary measure. Transformed cells are cloned in much the same manner as fused cells but if no pre-selection has been employed, many more plates should be used for each clone and it may be anticipated that the majority of clones will be negative so that a very wide screen will have to be used to detect positive clones.

8.4. Failure of cloning

8.4.1. Introduction

It is at the cloning stages rather than the fusion stages that most hybridomas are lost. Sometimes this is unavoidable as the clone loses the appropriate chromosome at an early stage of development where it has not been possible to freeze enough stocks. If the parent hybridoma has been maintained in culture however and if stocks have been frozen, it is possible to repeat the whole process with the same hybridoma. In cross-species fusions, chromosome loss is clearly a complex and selective process (Croce et al., 1980) with different human chromosomes being retained. Fusions between myeloma cells result in the retention of different chromosomes from fusions between fibroblasts. In intraspecies fusions such an analysis is difficult to perform although it is known that fusion of two differentiated cells of different types tends to lead to the suppression of differentiated functions. Consequently, it may be possible that a fusion which has occurred between the myeloma cell and a lymphocyte at an inappropriate stage of differentiation to match the myeloma will result in a clone that will always be unstable. Myeloma lines have been selected over the years to avoid this situation as far as possible. The practical experience of most laboratories is that a clone which ceases to secrete at early stages remains unstable if it is recloned.

8.4.2. Failure with no growth

Clones grow at very different rates according to the culture conditions and at least four weeks should elapse before they are discarded. Failure of this type usually indicates a reagent problem. The reagents can be tested by cloning the parent myeloma using identical procedures. In soft-agar cloning the agar can sometimes be found to be toxic or may have been mixed with the cells at too high a temperature. Any remaining cells of the parent hybridoma line should also be checked for contamination, particularly with mycoplasma. If the parent hybridoma is still positive then the cells should be recloned with a plate of parent myeloma cells as control.

8.4.3. Failure with clonal growth

It is quite common to have substantial clonal growth and very few wells positive. If this occurs in wells seeded at above 1 cell/well then an obvious explanation is that the required cells have been overgrown by others which secrete either no antibody or the wrong antibody. However, good growth can also occur at high dilution with little antibody production. This usually means that cloning was delayed for too long and that among those cells to be cloned there were in fact very few which secreted antibody of the appropriate specificity. Since non-producers are assumed to grow faster than producers (see Section 8.3.1 for discussion), earlier cloning would have led to a higher proportion of clones which secreted antibody of the chosen specificity. An alternative explanation is that the original clone was unstable and tended to lose the required chromosome (see Section 8.4.1). In either case, it is likely that the remaining cells of the parent hybridoma will no longer make significant amounts of antibody. Any positive wells should be expanded and subcloned again. If the same phenomenon occurs on second subcloning at 1 cell/well or lower then the hybridoma may never be very useful as it is clearly unstable. However, if the second subcloning is successful then future fusions should be assayed and cloned at earlier stages, or many more cloning plates should be used in order to increase the statistical changes of finding a positive clone.

8.5. Continuation of cloning

Most protocols suggest that two limiting-dilution subclonings are adequate to produce a fully monoclonal antibody producing hybridoma. It is, however, advisable to reclone hybridomas regularly in the first few months to test their stability. In particular it is essential to screen subsequent clonings for any clones with good growth but no antibody production as these indicate either that the original cloning was not adequate or that the hybridoma was unstable and will be difficult to grow in bulk culture with continued antibody production.

CHAPTER 9

Antibody production and purification

9.1. Maintenance of cell stocks

During the cloning procedures, hybridomas should have been frozen down at every stage. Once the hybridoma is established a large number of vials of fully cloned cells should be frozen and their ability to recover from liquid nitrogen checked. It is advisable to keep frozen vials in more than one nitrogen container in case of equipment failure as there may be periods of time when it is not convenient to propagate the parent line in culture. The antibody-producing cells should be recloned at least twice a year and checked regularly for mycoplasma contamination.

9.2. Expansion of hybridomas in vitro

Hybridomas are best expanded slowly in vitro by transfer to 24-well Costar plates followed by 25-cm^2 flasks, 80-cm^2 flasks and 175-cm^2 flasks with the cell density maintained between 10^5 and 10^6 cells/ml. At early stages some hybridomas grow very slowly and may be helped by the addition of feeder cells. As the hybridomas become established, the concentration of FCS can usually be slowly reduced to as low as 5%. Typical culture supernatants yield up to 100 µg/ml of antibody, the exact amount depending on the cell density and rate of growth. Human hybridomas or transformed cells give very low yields (1–2 orders of magnitude lower), the yield from transformed cells which have not been fused with a second myeloma after transformation being particularly poor.

If large amounts of antibody are required, it is best to set a flask aside for this purpose, grow the cells to exhaustion and discard them retaining the supernatant. The main cell line for propagation should always be in exponential growth. It should also be recloned regularly. Cells at this stage may be grown in gassed roller bottles if this is more convenient and saves incubator space.

Another convenient method for growing large amounts of hybridoma in tissue culture is by the apparatus shown in Fig. 9.1 (Techne). The cells are slowly stirred by the central shaft and medium may be added or removed from the side arms so that continuous culture is possible. Cells are grown in a 37° water bath and must be gassed regularly. Fazekas de St. Groth (1983) has described a method for automated production in a cytostat.

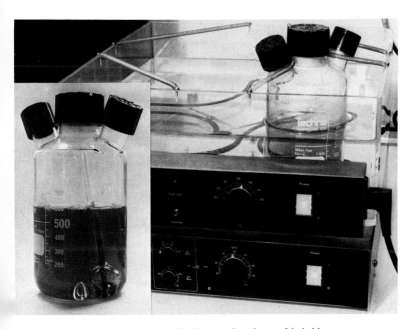

Fig. 9.1. An apparatus for large scale culture of hybridomas.

Large scale culture vessels have also been described (Galfre and Milstein, 1981) and apparatus for the production of 5 litre cultures may be purchased. However, if really large amounts of antibody are required it may be wiser to approach some of the Biotechnology companies such as Celltech, U.K. Ltd. who will grow bulk cultures to yield kilogram quantities of antibody. If this sort of amount of antibody is required then it must have commercial potential.

Culture in vitro provides a more pure preparation of antibody. The only protein contaminants are from the FCS which has up to 1.3 mg/ml bovine immunoglobulin (Underwood et al., 1983) but no contaminating rat, mouse or human immunoglobulin and which can be used at low concentrations on an established hybridoma. Contamination may be further reduced by the use of serum-free medium (Iscove and Melchers, 1978) or, for very-short-term cultures of 24 to 48 h, no medium at all. Nuclease and protease contamination is minimal.

Propagation in vitro is also the only effective method of growing some rodent hybridomas and most human hybridomas. While human hybridomas may in theory be propagated in nude (athymic) mice this procedure has a low success rate and such mice require special animal facilities for maintenance.

9.3. Expansion of hybridomas in vivo

Mice primed with mineral oils tend to be more susceptible to the development of spontaneous Mineral Oil induced PlasmoCytomas (MOPCs) and this fact is used to encourage hybridoma growth in vivo. The mice are primed by intraperitoneal injection of 0.5 ml pristane (tetramethylpentadecane) (Aldrich) 5–10 days before intra-peritoneal inoculation with 10^6 to 10^7 hybridoma cells. It is impor-tant to use mice which are histocompatible with the parent cells and thus if the original fusion was between myeloma cells of Balb/c origin and the mouse was NZB then the hybridoma should be propagated in a F1 hybrid of the two strains.

Hoogenrad et al. (1983) have shown that a 10-day interval between pristane priming and tumour injection gives maximal amounts of antibody in the tissue-culture fluid and also a high percentage of responding mice. However, the rate of growth of the resulting ascites tumours is in general very variable and can be from less than two to more than five weeks. If it takes a long time, then it is possible that the tumour may be a spontaneous one induced by the pristane. The fluid can be tapped from an anaesthetised mouse or removed from a dead one according to choice and the methods are given in Appendix 1. Frequently the hybridomas grow as solid tumours early on and are only established as free cells after several passages so it is probably best to kill the animal and inspect the peritoneal cavity after the first propagation. (Interestingly enough, residual mineral oil is often found in ascites tumours which grow at an early stage.) It is possible to obtain 10 ml of acites fluid or more from a mouse and 50 ml or more from a rat by regular tapping. Titres are variable and may be low early on but the amount of antibody in an established ascites line should be close to several milligram/ml. IgM-producing hybridomas are sometimes reported not to grow in ascites fluid but most do, although with a slightly lower titre.

At every passage the antibody production should be checked to ensure that no reversion to non-secretion has occurred. Ascites cells recover from freezing exceptionally well and can be frozen down in the same way as tissue-culture cells and reintroduced into animals without difficulty.

It is sometimes suggested that hybridomas can be propagated before full cloning but this is not likely to lead to successful hybridoma production in theory and does not do so in practice in the mouse. Rat hybridomas are more stable and may be amenable to such treatment.

Ascites fluid will be contaminated with mouse immunoglobulins to a small extent and if a very pure antibody is required this may prove inconvenient. Other protein contaminants are readily removed (Section 9.7) but immunoglobulins co-purify with most recommended techniques. Ascites fluid is also more likely to have protease and nuclease contamination.

As a general rule an antibody for laboratory use 'in house' cells can be usefully propagated in vivo. However, if a commercial reagent of proven record is required, it is probably more convenient to set up in vitro propagation systems. This is likely to remain a good rule as long as good large scale culture techniques develop at the current rate.

In vivo expansion with solid subcutaneous tumours (Galfre and Milstein, 1981) has also been used and is reported to be more easily managed than ascites propagation but is less frequently used.

9.4. Failure in expansion

If a cell line fails to grow readily in vitro despite having been subcloned at least twice then it should be expanded very slowly indeed with a highly restricted range of cell concentrations only diluting the cells 2–5-fold. Feeders may help at early stages but are impractical at later stages. Slow expansion will yield enough antibody for its true value to be tested and may allow the cells to adapt. Further subcloning to search for a more robust line is also an obvious option.

If ascites tumours fail to grow then the recipient mice may be irradiated at 300–400 R or nude mice may be used. Both types of mouse are susceptible to infection and should be maintained under germ-free conditions. The most likely source of ascites failure is histocompatibility difficulty and if persistent growth failure is experienced with several hybridomas it is wise to obtain a hybridoma known to grow in the strain of mouse which is being used and test it on the animals available or to obtain a fresh breeding stock of the correct pedigree. This problem has already occurred with the Lou rat line where the animals available in the U.K. are no longer suitable hosts for the original cell line developed by Bazin although they are suitable for the U.K. cell lines and comparable with the rats from U.K. suppliers such as Olac (Appendix 2) (Bazin, 1983). Occasional hybridomas which do not grow in vitro have been reported but it is not clear whether this is due to a genuine abnormality of the cell line or laboratory histocompatibility problems as most hybridomas should grow readily in this way.

If a cell line grows but the antibody secretion falls off it should be recloned immediately. Bulk production should not have been initiated unless full cloning was carried out and the most likely source of this difficulty is initial undercloning. However, a non-secreting mutant may arise at any time.

9.5. Storage of antibody

Polyclonal sera are usually extremely stable. This is traditionally supposed to be because of the large number of disulphide bonds which are present on immunoglobulins. Most monoclonal antibodies are also stable and can be frozen and thawed readily. It is, however, advisable to check the titre after freezing and thawing at an early stage as the storage of supernatant will be affected by such a susceptibility and it is customary to freeze fairly large amounts of supernatant before antibody purification is commenced. Many IgM antibodies do not retain full antigen-binding capacity after freezing and thawing but many do. In general, an antibody which does not freeze well, like one which does not grow or clone well, is better discarded unless it is of considerable importance in which case it should be stored in 0.1% sodium azide at 4 °C.

Monoclonal antibodies, like serum, should not be repeatedly frozen and thawed and it is best to freeze 4 or 5 small aliquots from each tissue-culture flask or ascites fluid tap separately from the bulk for general use or for testing before purification on a large scale.

9.6. Concentrating the antibody

Before concentrating a monoclonal antibody it may be helpful to ascertain its immunoglobulin class (Chapter 10). Most antibodies from ascitic fluid are already concentrated. However, antibodies from tissue-culture media can present a genuine problem if large amounts of culture medium have to be handled. This is particularly true with human hybridomas where the yield in tissue-culture medium is low. As in all other cases, a monoclonal antibody cannot be assumed to behave like bulk immunoglobulin but it is likely that it will do so and its properties in this respect can be tested on a small pilot batch at an early stage. Most immunoglobulins precipitate free from the main contaminating protein which is albumin at 40% saturation with ammonium sulphate (some antibodies require 50% which may mean a slight increase in contamination with other serum proteins) and can then be dissolved in a smaller volume, dialysed into PBS, assayed, and frozen or used for further purification.

Antibodies which cannot be partially purified in this manner may be concentrated by conventional means such as dialysis against a powder of hygroscopic material (most hybridoma laboratories use PEG for this purpose) to reduce the volume, by vacuum dialysis, or by filtration through selective membranes (Amicon). In any of these cases some antibody tends to be lost by sticking to the membranes or the dialysis tubing (which must not be allowed to dry out) or filter. However, if the antibody is still relatively impure, the other proteins in the FCS or ascites fluid protect against this to some extent.

The entire culture medium may also be lyophilised although this leads to a very high salt concentration. Dialysis before lyophilisation may lead to the precipitation of the particular antibody involved, especially if it is an IgM. Again a small pilot experiment is useful.

In principle, it is not necessary to concentrate a valuable antibody if it is fed slowly onto an affinity or Protein A column (see below). However, a few preliminary experiments may save much technical time.

9.7. Purification of the antibody

9.7.1. Introduction

In many cases purification of an antibody is not necessary since all that is required is specificity and each batch of antibody can be tested for titre and used directly. However, if a monoclonal antibody is required as a standard reagent, or for therapeutic purposes it must obviously be purified. In addition, many of the methods used to characterise a monoclonal antibody involve labelling it with either enzymes or isotopes and a pure antibody is obviously more suitable for this purpose. Likely, protein contaminants from tissue culture are proteins in the FCS. While these are largely albumins there may also be contamination with bovine immunoglobulin (Underwood et al., 1983) which may be removed by protein A. There may also be contamination with small amounts of soluble cellular debris which may include proteases and nucleases. In ascitic fluid, likely contaminants include irrelevant immunoglobulin which is less readily removed together with larger amounts of proteases and nucleases. The extent of contamination with irrelevant immunoglobulin also depends on the class of antibody. As with most other techniques involving monoclonal antibodies it is better to attempt small pilot purification experiments to see whether the antibody involved can be purified by the method which is contemplated.

A general concept which has been referred to before (Section 2.4) should be further emphasised. Low amounts of antibody are readily lost by non-specific adsorption to plastic surfaces. The antibody should not be transferred among innumerable containers before, during or after any purification procedure unless there is an excess of another protein present. In the case of purification, where the object is to remove other proteins, this can readily occur. Glass containers are less likely to adsorb antibody but may still do so in a solution of low concentration.

Before purification it is important to determine the class of the antibody (Chapter 10) as this will affect which procedure is used. As with all protein-purification techniques, antibodies may be separated according to charge or size. In addition, they may be purified by affinity chromatography utilising Protein A for certain types and species, by anti-immunoglobulin columns, or by antigen affinity columns if large amounts of antigen are available.

Immunoglobulin purification is covered extensively by many excellent books directed primarily towards the purification of immunoglobulin from serum samples (Weir, 1978; Johnstone and Thorpe, 1982). Conversely, some reviews and original papers are directed towards small and statistically insignificant groups of myelomas. These are extremely useful as general guides. However, where a protocol has been derived for serum in general, some of the steps may be unnecessary particularly in purification from tissue-culture fluid where there is little contaminating immunoglobulin and many of the procedures may be simplified. Where a protocol has been derived from experience with a limited number of hybridomas, of the relevant class, it may be followed experimentally with reasonable optimism, but persistent negative results may be due to variations in the antibody structure rather than technical inadequacy.

9.7.2. Purification with Protein A

The commonest reagent to be utilised in antibody purification is Protein A. This protein is synthesised by *Staphylococcus aureus* and binds to the Fc region of many IgG molecules (reviewed by Langone, 1982a,b). It is available at low cost from most commercial suppliers either alone or coupled to various matrices such as Sepharose (Pharmacia). Protein A is useful for the purification of IgG antibodies of most classes but is reported to be a poor adsorbant for IgG_3 in both mouse and human though the data are sparse because of the comparative rarity of IgG_3 myelomas and Kronvall et al. (1970) and Grey et al (1971) report the same myeloma line to be positive and negative respectively for Protein A binding. Additionally, evidence is accumulating to suggest that only certain allotypes of human IgG_3 can bind to Protein A (Haake et al., 1982). The situation with mouse IgG_1 is complex and may relate to the possibility of subdivision of this class of antibody (Stanislawski and Mitard, 1976). Mouse IgG_1 is frequently reported to bind Protein A in general textbooks. However Kronvall et al. (1970) reported that none of a selected group of IgG_1 antibodies bound. The binding properties vary with several parameters, and some authors have used differential pH (Kohler et al., 1978; Trucco et al., 1979) while others have used differential ionic strength in their estimation of affinity for Protein A. The general procedure developed by Ey et al. (1978) for serum samples is most commonly employed, and a parallel procedure for human serum has also been developed (Duhamel et al., 1979). There is also some dispute as to the effect of Protein A on rat IgG molecules but Ledbetter and Herzenberg (1979) found that only rat IgG_{2c} antibodies bound at pH 7 while some rat IgG_{2a} antibodies bound at pH 8.6. However, Rousseaux et al. (1981)

TABLE 9.1

Relative affinities of various IgGs for Protein A

Species		Reference
Mouse		
IgG_1	Low but some binding at pH 8	
IgG_{2a}	Medium	Ey et al. (1978)
IgG_{2b}	High	
IgG_3	Low	
Rat		
IgG_1	Medium	
IgG_{2a}	Very low	Rousseaux et al. (1981)
IgG_{2b}	Low	Nilsson et al. (1982)
IgG_{2c}	High	
Human		
IgG_1	High	
IgG_2	Medium	Duhamel et al. (1979)
IgG_3	Certain allotypes only	
Rabbit		
IgG	High	Goding (1976)
		Miller and Stone (1978)

found that the affinity in descending order was IgG_{2c}, IgG_i, IgG_{2b}, and IgG_{2a} with considerable difference in affinity among individual monoclonal antibodies of each separate class. Table 9.1 gives a summary of the available data to date. Nilsson et al. (1982) have published a detailed protocol for the purification of all classes of rat IgG from serum. It should be emphasised that serum analysis may not correlate with the properties of any particular monoclonal antibody.

IgM and IgA antibodies of all species do not in general bind to protein A although human IgA_2 may bind in some cases. However, the behaviour of no single monoclonal antibody can be predicted since the allotypic regions may contribute to alterations in binding properties. The only sensible course of action is to perform a small pilot experiment to ascertain the properties of the monoclonal antibody in question. Rabbit IgG appears to have a high affinity for protein A and may consequently be used in monoclonal 'sandwich' detection systems (Chapter 2).

Protocol 9.1
Pilot purification with Protein A (mouse antibodies)
   (i) Suspend 1 g of protein A-Sepharose CL-4B (Pharmacia) in 200 ml PBS pH 8.0 containing 0.1% sodium azide for at least 30 min. Use a small chromatography column (e.g. Pharmacia C10/10) or the barrel of a disposable 10-ml syringe plugged with a sintered glass filter. Pour the gel gently trying to leave no discontinuities and a final flat surface. The column can be run at room temperature. If it is to be stored it should at 4 °C and this may alter its flow properties. For a small column this is unimportant. Larger columns which will be re-used should be both poured and stored at 4°. Wash the column with at least 100 ml PBS + azide pH 8 followed by 100 ml 0.1 M sodium citrate pH 3 and re-equilibrate with PBS buffer pH 8.
   (ii) The tissue-culture supernatant used should have a titre of at least 1 in 100 so that comparisons between titre before and after purification may be made. The pH will probably already be in the order of 7.5 and should be made up to 8 by the addition of tris base or by dialysis into 10 mM tris HC1, 10 mM phosphate buffer pH 8

followed by centrifugation of any precipitate (which will probably be IgM and should be redissolved in culture medium and tested for antibody titre). A preliminary ammonium sulphate precipitation followed by dialysis into PBS pH 8 is best for large amounts of antibody provided that this is known to result in the retention of activity (Section 9.6).

(iii) Add 2 ml of the antibody to the column and allow it to flow in slowly. Wash with 5 ml 10 mM PBS pH 8 collecting 0.5-ml fractions of eluate (there should be no protein after 3–4 ml eluate). The quickest test is to blow a small amount of air through a pasteur pipette into the tubes to see if there is any froth indicating protein but a more scientific test is to monitor absorbance at 280 nm for proteins with aromatic amino acids or 230 nm for all proteins with a buffer with low UV absorbance. These intitial tubes should be kept for analysis. If they are strongly positive then the antibody does not bind to Protein A. If they are weakly positive then the column may have been overloaded. Wash the column with at least 5 ml of the same buffer. Most IgA, IgM and IgG_3 antibodies will be in this fraction but exceptions are possible.

(iv) Elute the column with 5 ml 0.1 M sodium citrate pH 6, taking 0.5-ml fractions. An IgG_1 antibody should be in this fraction. Before analysing these for immunological activity, either dialyse each into PBS or dilute with 10 × PBS until the pH and ionic strength are close to those normally employed for assay.

(v) Elute the column with 5 ml 0.1 M sodium citrate buffer pH 4.5 collecting 0.5-ml fractions. Treat the samples as in (iv). This fraction should contain IgG_{2a}.

(vi) Elute the column with 5 ml 0.1 M sodium citrate buffer pH 3.5 collecting 0.5-ml fractions as before. This fraction should contain IgG_{2b}.

(vii) If the column is to be recycled it should be washed at an even lower pH (50 mM citric acid is very effective) before being equilibrated with PBS + azide.

Note. If the antibody has been shown to have a high sensitivity to denaturation at low pH values by preliminary testing then it may be eluted using increasing salt concentrations as with affinity chromatography (Protocol 9.3).

9.7.3. Purification with DEAE-linked reagents

DiEthylAminoEthyl (DEAE) cellulose has been used for many years in the purification of IgG antibodies. More recently, variants comprising the DEAE group attached to acrylamide or beaded cellulose have become available. These give a much higher flow rate. Additionally QEAE compounds with a higher density of positive groups have become available attached to similar matrices.

The background to the use of positively charged ligands for IgG purification lies in the comparatively large numbers of basic amino acids present on the constant regions of most types of IgG. As a consequence of this, these immunoglobulins have poor binding to DEAE groups at low pH and at ionic strength values where most other serum proteins bind strongly. They can, therefore, be recovered in the early fractions of a gentle elution with an ionic strength gradient of a column of impure antibody bound with 10 mM phosphate buffer, pH 7.

While protein A is believed to react with aromatic residues, this technique relates to basic residues which are much more common and consequently there is less variability among species. However, murine IgGs have a much wider variation in the number of basic residues in the constant region of the immunoglobulin chain than most others and any particular hybridoma may behave abnormally on DEAE columns.

DEAE columns are frequently employed for the purification of IgG from other serum contaminants but are less well characterised with respect to the separation of IgG classes. With the antibody from a hybridoma this generally does not matter since there are few contaminating Igs of other classes. However, proteolytic or nucleolytic activities may copurify, particularly if ascites fluid is used as the starting material. Bruck et al. (1982) have tested DEAE-Affi Gel Blue columns with ascitic fluid from over 26 hybridomas as the starting material and find that by varying elution with respect to both pH and ionic strength, it is possible to eliminate both contaminants.

The main advantage of DEAE over Protein A is that extremes of pH are not necessary for purification as ionic strength gradients may be used. They are also economic and easy to work with and are available on a wide variety of matrices. An economic source is a microgranular cellulose from Whatman in the preswollen form DE52. However Pharmacia market DEAE sephadex, DEAE sepharose and DEAE sephacel according to whether the support for the ion exchanger is dextran, agarose or beaded cellulose all of which differ in cost, flow rate, binding capacity and ease of use. Bio-Rad market DEAE bound to beaded agarose and also DEAE Affi-Gel Blue which is claimed to bind all serum proteins with the exception of IgG and transferrin. Protocol 9.2 is given for DEAE-Sephacel which is easy to use and suitable for a pilot procedure. For scaling up to a production column other considerations such as cost or flow rate may be more important.

Protocol 9.2

Pilot purification of an IgG monoclonal antibody on DEAE Sephacel

(i) Dialyse either the antibody solution or an ammonium sulphate precipitate into 10 mM sodium phosphate pH 7.2. Some forms of mouse IgG are reported to precipitate with this procedure. Goding (1980) suggests that such precipitates be loaded onto the column. They may also be centrifuged free and redissolved and assayed.

(ii) Pour an 8-ml column of DEAE Sephacel (Pharmacia) in the barrel of a 10-ml pipette plugged with a sintered glass filter and equilibrate with 50 ml 10 mM phosphate pH 7.2. This will bind more than 1 g albumin which is the major contaminant in both culture medium and ascites fluid. The amount loaded may obviously depend on the extent of the albumin contamination which will be lower in an ammonium sulphate precipitate. The column should however not be overloaded with amounts of over 1 mg protein.

(iii) Run the solution into the column and wash with 10 ml 10 mM phosphate pH 7.2 collecting 1-ml fractions. Virtually all the protein should have bound. Form a gradient elution system by gradual mixing of 100 ml 10 mM phosphate pH 7.2 with 100 ml of the same buffer containing 0.2 M NaCl in the usual gradient procedure, collecting 1-ml samples. The IgG usually purifies in the fractions of NaCl concentration between 30 and 50 mM. Stepwise gradient elution with the NaCl concentration being raised in 20-mM increments is also effective for most IgGs.

(iv) Assay the samples and regenerate the column by washing with 10 ml guanidine hydrochloride followed by 50 ml of the original phosphate buffer.

9.7.4. Purification utilising affinity chromatography

Affinity chromatography is generally only used on antibodies which fail to purify with Protein A or DEAE techniques as it is less general a method. It is particularly useful in selecting minor components of a complex mixture and this is not the usual situation with hybridomas. Detailed descriptions of all possible procedures are given in the Pharmacia literature. The protocol given is for cyanogen bromide activated sepharose which is a relatively expensive method. Costs may be much reduced by preparing cyanogen bromide activated sepharose in the home laboratory rather than purchasing it. However, for pilot experiments it is probably more economical with respect to time to test the purchased material to see if the procedure is likely to be one which will be extensively employed. Methods for activating Sepharose with cyanogen bromide are given by Pharmacia literature and in standard texts (Johnstone and Thorpe, 1982).

Cyanogen bromide activated sepharose reacts with amino groups and is suitable for use with all antibodies directed against the Ig to be purified. If antigens are to be used in affinity purification then other types of sepharose reacting with groups which are not essential for coupling to the specific antibody may be more appropriate.

It is possible to purchase conventional anti-IgG antiserum or antibodies which are usually raised in one animal by the injection of the IgG of another with no further purification. Obviously, many of the antibody molecules in such serum will not be directed to the foreign IgG and less than 10 % will have the required specificity. 'Affinity purified' anti IgG samples which are also commercially available have been themselves pre-purified by affinity chromatography so that every antibody in the sample has the capacity to bind the IgG.

The antibodies which may be purchased for coupling include those directed against total mouse, rat or human IgG or (in the case of mouse and human antibodies) against a specific class of IgG. The latter type of antibody is expensive as its preparation is complex but will ensure that there is no contamination with antibodies of other IgG classes. It is of course more economical to prepare antibodies to mouse, rat or human IgG by immunising a rabbit, sheep or goat with the crude material. Again the recommended procedure is to purchase a fairly specific antibody for pilot work and consider production of this antibody in the home laboratory only if the procedure is to be used on a larger scale.

Protocols for the binding of immunoglobulins to CNBr-activated sepharose vary widely according to a variety of conflicting considerations. Coupling is more efficient at high pH but may lead to loss of antigenic activity if too many amino groups are bound per molecule. The protein concentration is also critical since too low a protein concentration may also lead to loss of activity because of over attachment. Ideally, only a small percentage of the added protein should be bound as this means that there will only be a few covalent attachment sites in each molecule. However, if too many antibody molecules are bound to the gel they may exhibit steric hindrance among their active sites and more high affinity sites which are hard to elute may be present. Protocol 9.3 is a rough guide. If higher pH values are used, more protein should be added because of the above considerations.

Protocol 9.3
Affinity purification of mouse IgG

(i) Weigh out 0.5 g CNBr-activated sepharose 4B and suspend in 10 ml 1 mM HCl. Wash with aliquots of 10 × 10 ml of 1 mM HCl on a sintered glass filter, porosity G3. Do not allow the gel to dry out.

(ii) Prepare 5 mg anti-mouse IgG (from sheep, goat or rabbit) in 1 ml 0.2 M NaHCO$_3$ buffer pH 8.3 containing 0.5 M NaCl (coupling buffer). Wash the gel with 2 ml coupling buffer and then *immediately* mix with the protein solution either at room temperature for 2 h or overnight at 4° using gentle stirring or shaking but not a magnetic stirrer which may damage the beads.

(iii) Add 0.2 ml 2 M ethanolamine or 0.2 M glycine pH 8 (blocking reagent) to block off reactive groups and mix gently for a further 1 h. Centrifuge at 500 g for 5 min and resuspend the gel in coupling buffer. Determine the amount of uncoupled antibody in the supernatant by ultraviolet absorption using a solution made up of the appropriate amounts of coupling buffer and blocking reagent as blank. A 1 mg/ml solution of most IgGs gives an absorbance of 1.35 at 280 nm. Less than 20 % of the antibody should have bound. The remainder may be precipitated with ammonium sulphate and reused.

(iv) Pour the gel into the barrel of a 5-ml disposable pipette plugged with a sintered glass disc. Wash with 50 ml coupling buffer and 50 ml 0.1 M sodium acetate pH 4. At this stage the column may be stored in PBS containing 0.1 % azide for a few weeks. However, even covalently bound protein slowly leaches off the column.

(v) Concentrate and partially purify the antibody to be used with ammonium sulphate precipitation if this does not destroy activity. Prepare a small pilot experiment on antibody dissolved in PBS at high titre. Take 4 tubes containing 0.1 ml of antibody. To the first add 1 ml 0.1 M glycine pH 2.5, leave for 10 min and neutralise with 2 M tris base (approximately 40 µl). To the second add 1 ml 0.1 M glycine buffer pH 10, leave for 10 min and add 1 M HCl (approximately 70 µl) to neutralise. To the third add 1 ml 3 M KSCN and to the fourth add PBS. Assay all 4 tubes (if the antibody titre is below 1 in 100 in the starting material, the antibody in KSCN should be dialysed first). This should give an indication of the possible sensitivity of the monoclonal antibody to possible elution procedures. If it is stable in all 4 then elution with low pH or high pH can be used for purification. However, with affinity purified antibody as the starting material it is sensible to use the eluting conditions employed for the preparation of this if the monoclonal antibody is stable under these conditions. If pH affects activity strongly then the chaotropic salt KSCN is more likely to be a suitable eluant although it is not convenient at low titres because of the need for preliminary dialysis of each fraction. A combination of pH and salt may be used on a very stable antibody for maximum elution. Elution with antigen may also be employed although this will affect subsequent assay procedures.

(vi) Pass 0.5 ml normal mouse serum through the column and elute with the chosen elution agent until no further protein is present in the eluate. This will saturate the very high affinity sites with irrelevant antibody.

(vii) Pour a 1-ml solution containing approximately 100–500 µg/ml of the ammonium sulphate precipitated antibody dissolved and dialysed into PBS onto the column. Run through slowly and wash the column with PBS until no further absorbance at 280 nm is detectable in the eluate. Elute with the chosen elution agent collecting 0.3–0.5 ml fractions. If changed pH has been used to facilitate elution then the fractions should be collected in tubes containing buffer which will return the pH of the eluted fraction to neutral as quickly as possible. Assay the eluted fractions and also the initial washes as this will give some estimate of the capacity of the column and the efficiency of the elution procedures.

9.7.5. Purification of an IgM monoclonal antibody

IgM monoclonal antibodies are most conveniently purified by precipitation at low ionic strength. Most IgM molecules will precipitate with dialysis into 2 mM phosphate buffer pH 6. The precipitate can then be centrifuged and washed with the same buffer and then resuspended in 10 mM tris/HCl, 0.15 M NaCl pH 7.2. As always, a small pilot experiment should be performed to ascertain that the antigenic activity is in this fraction. Contamination with IgG can frequently occur, especially in murine systems and the antibody should be further purified on a column of Sepharose 6B equilibrated with 10 mM tris/HCl pH 7.2, 0.15 M NaCl. While most pilot procedures involving affinity chromatography can be carried out in pasteur pipettes or the barrels of disposable syringes, separation which depends on size alone is best, even at pilot stage carried out on a proper chromatography column (e.g. Pharmacia C 10/10) since packing and correct flow rates are of greater significance. On Sepharose 6B, an IgM antibody should elute just behind the void volume which may contain aggregated material. IgG should be considerably retarded because of its low molecular weight. IgM can also be purified by affinity chromatography (Section 9.7.4) but is generally not successful in chromatography with Protein A- or DEAE-linked columns.

9.7.6. Purification of an IgA monoclonal antibody

IgA monoclonal antibodies are so rare that data on their purification is very sparse. Affinity chromatography is the only described technique which should prove reliable for all monoclonal antibodies of this class.

9.7.7. Failure of purification

Any monoclonal antibody of any class may exhibit characteristics which differ from the majority of antibodies in this class. It is easy to use this as an excuse for failure but such unusual antibodies are the exception and failure is more likely to be due to errors in technique.

Failure with either protein A or DEAE should be tested with other hybridomas or a polyclonal serum to ascertain the suitability of the reagents under normal conditions. The eluates should be checked with class-specific antiserum rather than antigen-specific assays. The conditions for elution should also be checked to make sure that they do not denature under the mild acidic conditions used for elution from Protein A or the low ionic strength used for loading on DEAE. Such preliminary checks are already incorporated in Protocol 9.3 for affinity chromatography in which elution conditions are more extreme.

Failure in affinity chromatography can be from several sources. Probably the most common one is in the difficulty in eluting the monoclonal antibody from the affinity column under conditions in which it does not denature. If all possible eluant combinations give denaturation or elution of no activity, then the column should be poured again with variation of the binding conditions. As already mentioned in Section 9.7.4 the affinity of the antibody may be altered either way by the number of binding sites on the bound antibody which are used in attachment to the insoluble matrix. It is very little extra effort to pour a small number of pilot columns under different conditions of protein concentration or pH. If the column was pre-saturated and pre-eluted under the same conditions with irrelevant immunoglobulin as recommended then it is most unlikely that the antibody has remained bound to the column. If the antibody was pre-tested for vulnerability to the elution conditions then it is unlikely to have been denatured. The most likely problem is therefore in the preparation of the affinity column.

CHAPTER 10

Characterisation of monoclonal antibodies

10.1. Introduction

The total characterisation of a monoclonal antibody is a long and complex procedure which varies widely with the intended use of the antibody. It is possible only to describe procedures relating to the characterisation of the monoclonality, and class in a volume this size although some indications of epitope specificity and general cross-reactivity may also be obtained from a few simple experiments. A general point which may be made however is that if a single hybridoma has been produced and is intended for a specific function it is unlikely that the antibody produced will have all the required characteristics. To produce monoclonal antibodies superior to conventional sera for most highly specialised functions it is better to make a large panel of cloned hybridomas and further select from these by characterisation of the antibodies they produce. This is clearly better performed at early stages and most of the techniques described are essentially small pilot ones which can be performed with small amounts of relatively impure antibody.

In contrast, however, it is a waste of both reagents and time to attempt full characterisation of an antibody which is not obtained from a fully cloned cell line. Most laboratories make no major attempt to determine antibody class until the hybridoma has been cloned twice. If an antibody of a certain class is specifically required (Sections 2.6.6 and 4.4) then methods of immunisation and selection should be altered.

10.2. Determination of antibody class

Antibody class is most readily determined by the use of class specific antibodies in an ELISA or by Ouchterlony assay. However, it is common also to use internally labelled antibody on polyacrylamide gel electrophoresis in both SDS and isoelectric focusing conditions. This is helpful in the determination of the relative proportions of the two antibody chains and in the case of isoelectric focusing, as final proof that the antibody is truly monoclonal. It is also helpful in the case of human hybridomas where the parent myeloma antibody and specific antibody chains are essentially competing for the protein synthesising machinery.

10.2.1. Class determination by ELISA

It is usual and frequently preferable to use a labelled second antibody directed to the whole IgG molecule (heavy and light chain) in an ELISA assay used for screening. This will detect most immunoglobulin classes because some of the epitopes will be on the lambda or kappa light chains even if they are not on the heavy chains. However, second antibodies labelled with most enzymes may also be obtained directed specifically to heavy chain determinants. Use of these antibodies in a conventional ELISA (Chapter 2) very readily determines whether the antibody is an IgM or IgG. However, labelled second antibodies directed against specific subclasses of IgG are not yet available. Unlabelled ones produced in rabbits are marketed by Miles and Nordic (Appendix 2) for the mouse and human systems. The class-specific anti-rat ones are produced in a variety of different animals for each class which is inconvenient. The quality of these reagents is variable and they should be tested extensively against serum on receipt so that the suppliers may be advised of deficiencies at early stages. In due course, when more competition among suppliers for chain-specific antibodies arises, the quality may improve.

In the case of a mouse antibody, the conventional ELISA is extended to include the IgG class-specific antibody with an enzyme-labelled sheep or goat anti-rabbit third antibody being used to produce the colour. Some cross-reaction frequently occurs due either to contaminating irrelevant IgG molecules in ascites fluid or possible cross-reactivity in the commercial material and it is important to titre either or both the monoclonal and the subclass-specific antibody across the plate in serial dilutions since at high concentrations reaction is likely to occur with all monoclonal antibodies of the IgG class and subclass-specific antibodies.

Antibody characterisation of this type is a classic example of a situation in which a polyclonal second antibody is actually preferable to a monoclonal one since it is desirable to have the antibody react with as many epitopes as possible. The ideal second antibody would be a well characterised and readily available mixture of monoclonal ones which could become a standard reagent and it is likely that commercial firms will produce such antibodies in the near future.

10.2.2. Class determination by Ouchterlony

Class determination by Ouchterlony analysis is probably the simplest method to use if the antibody is an IgG. It requires reasonable amounts of antibody to form a precipitate but takes little more than the ELISA with the extra 'sandwich'. It is undoubtedly less sensitive. Ouchterlony analysis is usually carried out on slides in solidified 1% agar (Difco) in which holes have been punched with a template to make a pattern of six outer wells and one inner. The agar is usually removed from the holes with a pasteur pipette by vacuum (for detailed procedures see Weir, 1978 or Johnstone and Thorpe, 1982). The polyclonal-specific antibody and the monoclonal antibody only form a precipitate under conditions in which neither is in excess. One slide is made for each of the four types of IgG and two sets of template are punched on each slide. In one set 10 µl of the hybridoma supernatant (or a redissolved ammonium sulphate fraction) is placed in the middle with doubling dilutions of class-specific antibody around the outside and in the other the (undiluted) class-specific antibody is placed in the centre with doubling dilutions of the hybridoma supernatant round the outside. The slides are incubated for 24 h at room temperature in a plastic box with damp tissues on the bottom to create a humidified atmosphere. The precipitate of monoclonal and class-specific antibody is seen as a thin white line between the central and outer wells.

If no precipitate is seen after 48 h, the sensitivity of detection can be greatly improved by staining the slide with Coomassie Blue (Section A.3.3). Failure to detect lines at this point indicates that equivalence has not been obtained and that either antibody or antigen (hybridoma antibody) were in excess and a different set of dilutions is necessary. Non-precipitating antibodies are unlikely to be present in this particular system unless a monoclonal second antibody has been used by mistake.

10.2.3. Class determination by electrophoresis of antibody labelled in vivo (Fig. 10.1)

Internally labelled antibodies run on polyacrylamide gels containing sodium dodecyl sulphate (SDS PAGE) give an indication of antibody class but do not permit subdivision of IgG antibodies into subclasses. The procedure involves the incorporation in vivo of radioactive amino acids into the monoclonal antibody by the hybridoma. It is usual to determine both cytoplasmic and secreted antibody since many myeloma and hybridoma lines exhibit considerable differences in their capacities to make and secrete the antibody. The main difference among protocols relates to the choice of labelled amino acid for this purpose.

Almost any amino acid may be used but Galfre and Milstein (1981) report that lysine, arginine and phenylalanine are incorporated into the myeloma protein of MOPC 21 at particularly high efficiency and this observation can be extrapolated to most IgG molecules on the basis of their isoelectric point and protein A binding capacity. Leucine is also commonly used. However the amino acid most frequently used for labelling is methionine. Amino acids can be obtained with ^{3}H, ^{14}C or (in the case of methionine) ^{35}S or ^{75}Se labels. The most economical

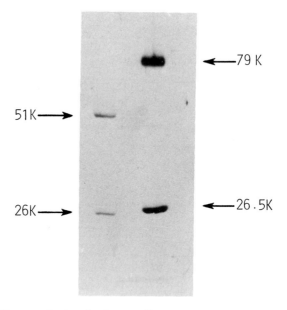

Fig. 10.1. Fluorograph of antibodies with ^{35}S-labelled methionine in vivo and then SDS_PAGE. Left, a monoclonal IgG; right, a monoclonal IgM. (Courtesy of A. Shallal.)

is ^{3}H which suffers the drawback of being a very weak β-emitter. [14]C amino acids are the most expensive. ^{75}Se-labelled methionine is reported to bind non-specifically to components of FCS (Gutman et al., 1978) although it has the advantage of being a γ-emitter. The most popular choice for labelling is ^{35}S-methionine which emits β-particles of approximately the same energy as ^{14}C and is cheaper and readily obtained at high specific activity. If the antibody is to be used only for class determination then ^{3}H-labelled amino acids may readily be used. However, for further extended use in competition assays (Section 10.4.1) or in tissue localisation, it may be less suitable. One drawback of ^{35}S-methionine is the relatively short half-life of methionine (87 days). This is quite long enough for most characterisation studies but could be inconvenient if very long-term use is envisaged.

In order to label the protein it is necessary to have the cells growing in medium which has very little non-radioactive amino acid. Commercial supplies of medium without any particular amino acid are readily obtained. Some procedures advise the dialysis of the FCS into PBS as well but the amino acid concentration in FCS is usually small (of the order of 10 mg/l) and if FCS is used at low concentrations it will not dilute the label significantly. Some protocols recommend labelling at high specific activity for a short period of time without any FCS present. If the specific activity of the amino acid is too low then very little will be incorporated into the monoclonal antibody. However, if the specific activity is so high as to make the amount of the amino acid a rate-limiting step in protein synthesis, then incorporation will also be poor and some protocols therefore recommend the addition of medium with 10% (around 3 mg/l) of the usual amino acid concentration of the medium, particularly where the hybridoma is making large amounts of antibody. If the cells are growing well and making antibody, these are the only main factors which will affect incorporation.

Protocol 10.1

Labelling in vivo of monoclonal antibodies with ^{35}S-methionine

Note. Observe the usual precautions required for working with radioactive samples.

(i) Obtain sheep anti-rabbit and rabbit anti-mouse antiserum and establish conditions under which precipitation equivalence is optimal in high detergent buffer (See (v)). Grow the hybridoma cells exponentially at a density of below 5×10^5 cells/ml. Before labelling check that viability is greater than 90%. At the same time, it is helpful though not essential to grow the parent myeloma line and marker cell lines known (and checked in the home laboratory) to secrete IgM, IgG and IgA under the same conditions and treat them in the same way as the hybridoma cells throughout the protocol.

(ii) Wash an aliquot of 5×10^5 cells in 5 ml RPMI minus methionine in a sterile conical universal. Centrifuge at 500 g and decant supernatant. Tap the pellet to loosen the cells and add 0.1 ml RPMI minus methionine medium containing 5% FCS and 100 μCi of ^{35}S-labelled methionine at 37° (800 Ci/mmole, Amersham).

(iii) Incubate at 37° in a humidified CO_2 incubator shaking at 15-min intervals to resuspend the cells. After 30 min, remove 50 μl and transfer to 2 ml ice-cold RPMI. Return then the remainder of the culture to the incubator. Centrifuge then sampled material at 500 g for 5 min, discard the supernatant, and resuspend the pellet in 2 ml 0.1 M Tris HCl pH 8, 0.1 M KCl, 0.005 M $MgCl_2$. When the cells are completely resuspended add 50 μl Triton X-100 in the same buffer and mix for 10 min. Centrifuge at 500 g for 10 min to pellet nuclei. Decant supernatant, discarding the pellet, and add 50 μl 10% sodium deoxycholate, 5% SDS in the same buffer. The radioactivity in this material represents the amount of antibody synthesised by the cell. Aliquot in 100-μl batches and store the material in eppendorf tubes at 4° until the material from step (iv) is ready for analysis.

(iv) 3–5 h after the start of the incubation, add 350 μl of cold RPMI and centrifuge at 500 g for 5 min. Decant the supernatant into an eppendorf tube containing 10% Triton X-100, 10% sodium deoxycholate and 5% SDS all dissolved in 0.1 M Tris HCl, 0.1 M KCl, 0.005 M $MgCl_2$. Discard the pellet. The radioactivity in this fraction represents the secreted antibody.

(v) Precipitate both synthesised and secreted antibody with rabbit anti-mouse antibody followed by goat or sheep anti-rabbit antibody. (Both second and third antibody should be in slight excess and a small pilot experiment with the particular antibodies used in the home laboratory will indicate what relative concentrations give a detectable precipitate in the same buffer and detergent solutions, see (i).)

(vi) At this stage the samples may be frozen at $-70°$ before analysis by SDS–PAGE and autoradiography (Appendix 3) or fluorography.

Notes. (i) The two samples of cellular and secreted antibody may be run on SDS–PAGE electrophoresis, stained and autoradiographed without further purification. The background with the stained secreted proteins should be low and the appropriate bands may be detected. The cytoplasmic antibody may, however, be contaminated with other proteins. This should be minimised by the immune precipitation procedure recommended in (v).

(ii) In theory only a second antibody should be necessary for immune precipitation. This is true also in situations where Ouchterlony analysis (Section 10.2.2) has established a defined range of second antibody which will cause precipitation. In practice it is quicker to use a third antibody known to precipitate the second one under defined conditions since the exact amount of antibody synthesised by the hybridoma under the incubation conditions may be variable.

10.2.4. Light-chain analysis

In the mouse, most antibodies carry the kappa light chain. In human systems it is often useful (Chapter 7) to know the type of light chain, especially if the cells are to be fused with mouse cells. While the procedure is essentially the same as that used for the heavy chains, differences due to glycosylation are particularly evident in light chains on SDS–PAGE because of the greater resolution of mobility.

Failure to obtain any radioactivity from the hybridoma on the autoradiography may be due to:

(i) The methionine being of the wrong specific activity. This problem is discussed above and if controls of myelomas or hybridomas of known secretion ability have been included at the same cell density and pre-tested for secretion (see i) it is unlikely to be a major difficulty. Control hybridomas are preferable as myelomas which do secrete, tend in general to have much higher secretion rates. If the control cell lines are positive then check that the hybridoma still has activity against the antigen with the usual assay. The clone used may have ceased to secrete.

(ii) The second or third antibodies may not precipitate the first. As long as the second antibody is precipitated by the third in a bulk experiment or an Ouchterlony analysis this should not be a difficulty. This is best tested by running the unprecipitated myeloma supernatant on SDS–PAGE electrophoresis to check that radioactivity is actually being incorporated into the antibody.

(iii) There are more antibody chains than expected on PAGE–SDS electrophoresis. The most obvious interpretation of this phenomenon is that the antibody is not correctly cloned and this is the usual interpretation in most cases. However, it has been observed (Kohler et al., 1978) that dual antibody secretion can occur in the mouse system. Differential glycosylation is one obvious possible cause of this and further resolution may be obtained by using labelled sugars for further analysis. This is more commonly observed with light chains because of their greater mobility.

Antibodies may also be labelled by procedures for the preparation of iodine-labelled second antibody (Johnstone and Thorpe, 1982). This is less satisfactory for class determination as it gives no indication of the relative rates of synthesis and secretion of the two chains.

10.3. Proof that the antibody is monoclonal

Determination of antibody class does not constitute final proof that an antibody is monoclonal. For some of the more sophisticated uses of monoclonal antibodies this is essential. While it is likely that there is only one cell type if the antibody produced can be shown to be only of the IgM class, it remains possible that there are two or more IgM-secreting hybridomas in the culture. An isoelectric focusing gel is the only final method of proof (Appendix 3). For this, internally labelled antibodies produced by Protocol 10.1 are focused and auto-radiographed. A single family of bands indicates that the antibody is monoclonal. Iodine-labelled second antibodies are poorly suited to this analysis since iodination may differentially alter the properties of the various molecules.

10.4. Epitope analysis

The most relevant aspects of epitope analysis relate to the final use of the monoclonal antibody produced. In general, however, one of the earliest questions which is asked of a panel of hybridomas is the extent to which they are directed at the same or at different epitopes.

This enables selective expansion of only those antibodies which have different determinants and can save much tissue-culture time. Analysis of cross-reactivity between the antigen and other similar antigens to determine the specificity of the antibody is usually required early in the analytical process. A requirement which often overlaps with this is the analysis of carbohydrate determinants since these tend to be present on a variety of different antigens and may lead to unexpected cross-reactivity. Where a complex mixture of antigens is to be dissected, the Western blot analysis is of particular value.

10.4.1. Determination of overlapping epitopes

Redundancy among a panel of monoclonal antibodies is usually quite high and is best detected early in screening. If a successful first fusion has led to the production of a monoclonal antibody to one epitope and it is necessary to determine which supernatants from among a second panel of hybridomas exhibit a different specificity then a competition assay based on the use of a labelled monoclonal antibody is fairly readily performed (Fig. 10.2). The exact method employed depends on the assay system used and the nature of the label on the antibody. Plates with attached iodine-labelled antibodies may be directly autoradiographed, whereas those with antibodies labelled with β-emitters the wells must be excised and the radioactivity determined separately. Assays based on simple nitrocellulose blots of antigen are particularly well suited to excision of the spots and liquid scintillation counting.

The exact epitope concentration on the antigen is generally unknown and clearly relevant in a competition assay. If there are many epitopes then both the unlabelled and the labelled antibody can bind without any competition occurring. For this reason the normal assay should be set up with doubling dilutions of hybridoma supernatant over a thousand-fold range of doubling dilutions (11 samples). Each sample is incubated with hybridoma supernatant and then with the second labelled hybridoma antibody. The samples are washed in the usual way and then counted. If the competition has occurred, then

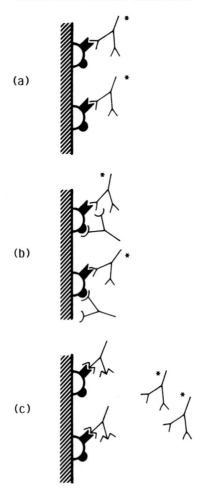

Fig. 10.2. Direct competition between labelled and unlabelled monoclonal antibodies. (a) The labelled antibody is bound directly to the solid phase antigen. (b) A second unlabelled antibody directed to a different determinant fails to compete and the bound radioactivity remains unchanged. (c) A second unlabelled antibody directed to the same determinant displaces the first (labelled) antibody and the level of bound radioactivity is decreased.

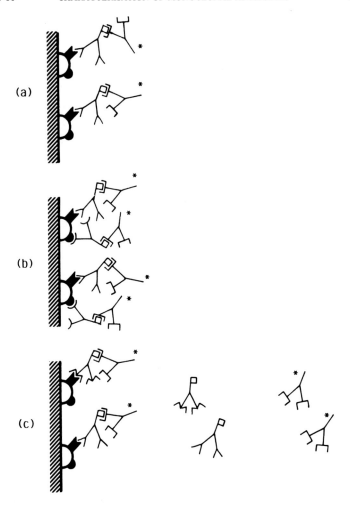

Fig. 10.3. Competition between two unlabelled monoclonal antibodies using a radioactive or enzyme-linked detecting antibody. (a) The reaction system with a single monoclonal antibody. (b) Competition with a second monoclonal antibody directed to a different determinant. The amount of detecting antibody bound to the solid phase is increased. (c) Competition with a second monoclonal antibody directed to the same determinant. The amount of detecting antibody bound is not increased.

at the highest concentration of unlabelled hybridoma supernatant, there should be few counts while at the lowest there should be a substantial number. Lack of competition is indicated by the same level of radioactivity throughout the dilution range. An important control to include is one containing dilutions of the unlabelled monoclonal antibody competing with its in vivo labelled counterpart to ensure that the experimental system is working. Friguet et al. (1983) have published an ELISA method for the analysis of overlapping epitopes which can be readily performed by the normal screening techniques (Fig. 10.3).

Positive competition in this system indicates that the labelled antibody and hybridoma supernatant share the same epitope, that their binding sites are so close together that the two cannot bind at the same time or that the binding of one causes a steric alteration in the antigen prohibiting the binding of the second. Lack of competition indicates either that the epitopes are distinct or that the hybridoma supernatant contained too little antibody to give effective competition.

10.4.2. Determination of antibody specificity among a group of antigens

The most obvious way of performing this particular task is to assay the antibody independently on each antigen and this is indeed the usual method of screening where antigens on material such as tissue sections are involved. However, most of the assays employed for hybridoma work are developed on ELISA systems, frequently with binding of the antigen to a solid matrix such as a microtitre plate. In this situation, difficulties in the comparison of antigens can arise due to differential binding to the solid matrix and the better assay which is also frequently the more convenient one involves competition between the two antigens (Fig. 10.4). The ELISA assay is set up as described in Chapter 2. The hybridoma supernatant is then pre-incubated for an hour at room temperature with the competing antigen before the solution of antibody and competitor are added to the plate. The assay is continued in the same way as a normal screening ELISA.

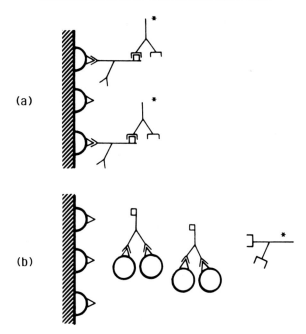

Fig. 10.4. Antigen competition ELISA. In (b) the free antigen competes with the plate bound antigen so that the bound signal is reduced.

An essential control is one incorporating the plate-bound antigen as a competitor. The concentration should range from no competitor to values exceeding the amount of plate bound antigen through a range of dilutions. Competition is indicated by a low ELISA reading at the higher concentrations of competing antigen. This technique is also particularly valuable in the quantitative analysis of determinants which may be present in variable amounts on different antigens.

Competition at the same level as that exhibited by the plate-bound antigen indicates that the determinant is present at a similar level on the competitor. No competition indicates that the determinant is absent or inaccessible. Intermediate competition indicates a reduced amount or reduced accessibility of the determinants on the competitor.

10.4.3. Analysis of epitope specificity by antigen modification

In principle, antigenic specificity may be analysed by modification of any of the amino acid residues on the antigen in the same manner in which enzymes are inactivated with standard reagents to analyse their active sites. This can give information relating to the amino acid residues involved in the structure of the determinant. However, this is of comparatively small value in the analysis of cross-reactivity among antigens. The analysis of carbohydrate epitopes is on the other hand frequently relevant in hybridoma technology. This is because, being highly antigenic, these tend to predominate in a fusion with glycoprotein and glycolipid antigens. There are a limited number of carbohydrate residues found on such antigens and epitopes analysis can give a good indication of whether potential cross-reactivity involving these residues may be likely.

One line of approach in the analysis of carbohydrate epitopes is to perform the usual ELISA in the presence of either sugars or lectins which bind to specific carbohydrates. Negative results in this type of assay are not necessarily indicative of a non-carbohydrate epitope since the sugar may have a particular conformation on the protein which differs from that of the free sugar. An alternative approach is to use chemical or enzymic reagents to alter the glycosidic residues. Periodate oxidation at low concentrations (10 mM) and neutral pH will modify only sialic acid residues. At 50 mM concentrations and pH 3 it will modify most other carbohydrate residues which have cis-hydroxyl groups. The altered antigen can then be used in a competition assay (Section 10.4.2) to determine whether it competes as effectively as the unmodified antigen. The enzymes used to remove carbohydrate include neuraminidase, galactose oxidase (Sigma, Koch-Light), and endoglycosydase H (Miles). Failure of these enzymes to remove antigenic activity does not indicate that the epitope is not at least in part carbohydrate but they provide comparatively simple methods for eliminating from the panel those antibodies which are specifically directed to a sugar residue and likely to cross-react among a large number of antigens.

If the antigen is a complex mixture of proteins then a competition assay among partially purified fractions of this mixture may also quickly eliminate antigens of no interest. If the antigen is a purified protein then partial digestion with trypsin, chymotrypsin, or cyanogen bromide followed by gel filtration chromatography can provide fragments for use in a competition assay or direct assay (Pierschbacher et al., 1981). However, antigenic sites are frequently composed of complex structures created by the juxtaposition of two or more residues which are distant from each other on the primary structure of the molecule and consequently a negative result from part of a molecule does not indicate that the determinant or part of the determinant is not present.

10.4.4. Analysis of epitope specificity by Western blot

A Western blot, in common usage, refers to the electrophoresis of the antigen followed by its subsequent transfer to nitrocellulose paper and incubation with specific antibody and then with labelled second antibody. The name originates from the use of Southern blots (Southern, 1965) for the analysis of DNA fragments on gels by labelled RNA probes and ensuing development of a system for the analysis of RNA fragments on gels with labelled DNA probes called 'Northern' blotting, and has no political or climatic origins. Western blotting was originally developed by Towbin et al. (1979) with polyclonal antiserum and has proved an exceptionally valuable tool in hybridoma technology (Clark et al., 1982; Yurchenko et al., 1982). However, it is technically very much harder to perform than Southern or Northern blots. These involve nucleic acids which have a standard charge density and can be separated readily by electrophoresis. A denatured antigen is actually required for reaction with the nucleic acid probe. With proteins which carry highly variable charges, electrophoresis is usually carried out in gels containing SDS or urea and these denature the antigen which may therefore not react subsequently with the antibody probe. The antigen may renature during the transfer to the nitrocellulose paper allowing the antibody-combining site to reform but the efficiency of this procedure may be low. Alternatively, the determinant may be a simple one whose structure is reactive in the unfolded primary structure of the antigen. The general specificity of such epitopes may be low.

Western blotting may be performed on two possible matrices. Most successful work has been performed on the conventional nitrocellulose matrix. The antigenic proteins will attach firmly but not covalently to this. An attractive alternative is the use of diazotized aminobenzyloxymethyl (DBM) paper to which the proteins are bound covalently. The paper with the attached antigens may thus be reused several times. While in theory this would appear to be an ideal system for screening the antibodies of hybridomas, particularly those raised against a complex antigenic mixture, the technology is extremely difficult. Complex and specific determinants may not be detected, comparatively large amounts of antibody are required, and the reusability of the DBM paper is limited by its extreme fragility.

Protocol 10.2 gives the general procedure for transfer of antigens to a paper support followed by their detection by blotting. In this protocol the use of an enzyme-linked second antibody is recommended and blotting to the more readily used nitrocellulose is suggested. If the procedure is successful then it is possible to expand it to the use of DBM paper. An enzyme-linked second antibody gives a quicker result, is more convenient and is advised where an ELISA is generally used for testing the antibody activity. If a radiolabelled second antibody is generally used in the laboratory then it may as easily be used for the Western blot. The choice of electrophoretic system is important because of considerations relating to denaturation and if possible, this should be varied.

Protocol 10.2

Western blot of one-dimensional gel

(i) Perform a spot test (Chapter 2) on nitrocellulose using a series of dilutions starting at 100% of the material to be subjected to electrophoresis. Ideally, if a denaturant is to be used in the gel, the antigen should be dissolved in this. Take this material through all the washing and staining procedures described in the protocol below. This can be performed at the same time or prior to the main experiment. Electrophorese the antigen, antigenic mixture, or partial digest of antigen by SDS–PAGE, PAGE alone, urea–PAGE or two-dimensional PAGE. It is sensible to start with simple PAGE and progress to the others to ensure that the system is working. If confidence is lacking use an antigen and antibody system known or likely to blot such as a polyclonal anti-BSA raised in the same species, utilising all the same reagents before employing the actual test antigen. Remove a slice of gel for staining after transfer.

(ii) Set up the electroblot system shown in Fig. 10.5. The procedure

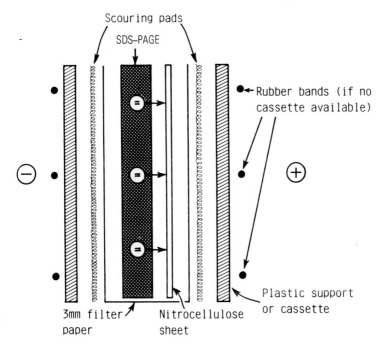

Fig. 10.5. Western blot apparatus for SDS_PAGE. Note that the apparatus is spread out for diagrammatic purposes and in use it is essential to have close and even contact between nitrocellulose and gel. SDS_PAGE is the polyacrylamide gel itself.

is slightly variable in that special blotting apparatus is now marketed (Biorad) whereas in the past the procedure was usually undertaken in an electrophoretic destaining apparatus. It is particularly valuable to have cooled apparatus for high voltages or long transfer periods as this will minimise the diffusion of the bands. The nitrocellulose sheet should be of 0.45 μ pore size (Millipore or Schleicher and Schull) and should be on the anode side of the gel if transfer is from SDS gels (i.e. the proteins are negative and likely to move to the anode). If urea gels at low pH are to be blotted, the paper should be on the cathode side of the gel. The apparatus remains the same but the electrodes are reversed. The nitrocellulose sheet should be wetted briefly before use. It is important not to allow any bubbles to form between the nitrocellulose sheets and the gel and the use of a folded sheet of Whatman 3mm paper around both gel and nitrocellulose minimises the chances of this. Secure the apparatus tightly with rubber bands (or pack it firmly into the cassette provided with the commercial apparatus) and place vertically in the electrophoresis chamber.

(iii) Transfer electrophoretically in 25 mM Tris HCl, 192 mM glycine pH 8.3 containing 20% v/v methanol and 0.002% SDS. For urea gels the transfer buffer is 0.7% acetic acid. The recommended voltage gradient is 6 V/cm/h (Towbin et al., 1979) but higher voltages may be used, preferably with some form of cooling system. The exact time required for transfer depends on the percentage of the acrylamide gels and the size of the protein to be transferred. Proteins above 100 000 in molecular weight are particularly difficult to blot unless they are in low percentage gels. For the first experiment a time of 2 h for a protein of molecular weight 50 000 in a 10% gel is a reasonable guide.

(iv) Switch off the power and remove the nitrocellulose sheet. Cut off a small strip for staining. Stain the slice of gel removed before blotting in (i) and the rest of the gel after blotting with Coomassie Blue (Appendix 2). Stain the nitrocellulose strip with 0.1% amido black in 10% v/v acetic acid, 45% v/v methanol. Destain with 70% v/v methanol, 4% v/v acetic acid. Coomassie blue is not a good stain for nitrocellulose as it is hard to destain. Incubate the remainder of the sheet with shaking for 2 or more hours in 50 mM Tris HCl, 150 mM

NaCl, 3% BSA, 5% adult sheep, goat or bovine serum and 0.05% sodium azide pH 7.4 to block off all the remaining sites (see also the note).

(v) Take a further unstained strip of the nitrocellulose paper to treat separately as a control. This should be treated in exactly the same manner as the experimental paper except that it should be incubated with similar tissue-culture medium to that in which the monoclonal antibody is contained. Incubate the blocked off paper for 4–16 h with the monoclonal antibody in 50 mM Tris HCl, 150 mM NaCl, 3% BSA, 0.05% azide pH 7.4 with shaking. This is most effectively performed in a polythene bag of the same size as the paper and makes optimal use of the antibody. The monoclonal antibody should have a titre of at least 1 in 100 in ELISA or radioactive binding assay. At the end of the incubation the antibody solution may be retained and is frequently reuseable.

(vi) Wash the nitrocellulose sheet several times with shaking in 50 mM Tris HCl, 150 mM NaCl pH 7.4. Then incubate with peroxidase-labelled anti-mouse antibody (for most commercial preparations dilute 1 in 100 or use the concentration most suitable from an ELISA determination) for 1 h at room temperature. Ideally, this should be affinity purified but few affinity purified conjugates are commercially available. Wash the nitrocellulose at least three times in 50 mM Tris HCl, 150 mM NaCl pH 7.4.

(vii) Incubate the nitrocellulose sheet in the dark for approximately 10 min with the substrate. The incubation solution is made up by mixing a stock of 3 mg/ml 4-chloro-1-naphthol in methanol with PBS in a ratio of 1:5 and adding H_2O_2 to 0.01% and should be freshly made up just before incubation.

(viii) Bands of a bluish colour should appear on the nitrocellulose corresponding to the antigen bands. The paper should be washed with distilled water and dried gently between leaves of Whatman 3mm filter paper and stored in the dark. The colour fades gradually over a period of weeks and the paper should be photographed within a week or so. The bands can be compared with the original gel or the stained paper but differential shrinkage usually occurs making detailed comparison difficult.

Note. In step (iv) BSA is recommended for blocking. However Batteiger et al. (1982) have shown that 0.05% Tween 20 may be used to block the nitrocellulose sheets instead of a protein such as BSA. This confers the considerable advantage of making it possible to stain the paper for protein after immunoblotting so that a very detailed comparison of the immunoreactive proteins may be obtained without the problems associated with differential paper shrinkage and gel expansion. See Addendum.

10.4.5. Failure to Western blot

The procedure outlined in Protocol 10.2 carries a number of controls which help to analyse difficulties which may occur at various points in the procedure.

(a) If no antigen has left the gel this will be clear from the staining of the gel before and after blotting. The small molecular weight antigens move more readily and it is common to find that these have blotted while the larger ones have not. In this case higher voltage or longer times are required. The gel concentration may also be reduced.

(b) If the antigen has left the gel but does not appear on the stained nitrocellulose strip then the electrodes may be of the wrong polarity, the contact between the gel and nitrocellulose may have been poor or the electrophoresis may have been for such a long period that the antigen has actually been electrophoresed into the paper and out of it again. The first two are the more common problems.

(c) If the antigen has left the gel, and the chemical staining of the paper shows that it is present there but there is no immunological stain then the antigen may be one which will not react because the epitope has been destroyed by the electrophoresis. Alternatively the concentration of the monoclonal or the second antibody may be too low. The efficiency of the second antibody can be checked by blotting of a standard protein as suggested in (i) with a polyclonal serum or by the recommended spot test. There is no set concentration that can be recommended for the monoclonal antibody but it is worth trying higher concentrations (Western blotting is very much less sensitive than ELISA) before concluding that the antigen does not respond because of irreversible denaturation. While the spot test is a good indicator of reagent quality, the antigens are not separated on it with the subsequent independent renaturation which occurs on electroblotting. It is possible at this stage to attempt to blot from a gel which involves less drastic denaturation.

(d) Sometimes more bands are stained than expected for a monoclonal antibody. This may of course be because the antibody has not been properly cloned. It may also be because of non-specific reaction of the antigens with the second antibody. This can be ascertained by examination of the strip of paper taken through the entire procedure but not incubated with the monoclonal antibody. Non-specific staining of this type is quite common, particularly if irrelevant IgG has not been incubated as recommended at step (iv). If the control strip is negative and there are still multiple bands on the experimental sheet then this may be either because the epitope has lipid and/or sugar or because it is genuinely polymorphic. Proteolysis is more common. A rare possible explanation for the appearance of an inexplicable extra band is peroxidase activity in the antigen itself.

(e) It is quite common to find a band on the paper which reacts with the antibody but has no counterpart in the original gel or stained paper. This may often be due to differential shrinkage making detailed comparison difficult but is also quite usual if a sensitive system has been used and indicates only that the antigen is a minor component of the mixture which has been subjected to electrophoresis.

10.4.6. Variations in Western blotting

Variations of this technique are numerous but the major ones relate to the type of paper and the techniques used for antigen detection. DBM paper is not recommended for initial work for the reasons discussed in Section 10.4.4. If it is required, then it may be purchased (Schleicher and Schull). Alternatively it may be made by techniques well covered in other texts (e.g. Johnstone and Thorpe, 1982).

Many experimental procedures involve the use of radiolabelled second antibodies. These have several disadvantages. Few suitable ones are commercially available and the radiolabelling must usually be performed in the home laboratory. This involves special controls, facilities and monitoring procedures in the U.K. and a great deal of extra time. The enzyme procedure yields results over a 24-h period while autoradiography or scintigraphy takes longer. However, the result is often clearer. It is also possible to label affinity purified antibody which should be superior to most enzyme-labelled ones. The quality of the labelled second antibody is highly variable in both techniques so that within any laboratory claims for superiority of enzyme- or isotope-labelling are also highly variable. However, some of the most elegant results with monoclonal antibodies have been obtained by the use of labelled Protein A (e.g. Yurchenko et al., 1982). This can be obtained labelled commercially (New England Nuclear). It can also be used to test conventional rabbit antiserum and then with mouse, rat or human hybridomas provided that an extra incubation with a second rabbit anti-IgG species-specific antibody is incorporated into the protocol before the addition of the labelled protein A (see Section 9.7.2 for Protein A specificity). Labelled Protein A should not be used directly on the monoclonal antibody unless its class and Protein A binding capacity have been ascertained.

Another useful variation on the blotting technique involves the electrophoresis of partial digests of the antigen to localise epitopes (Clark et al., 1982).

Several possible peroxidase substrates may be used for blotting and many commercial ones such as Biorad HRP colour development substrate are claimed to be superior by the makers.

Antibodies may also be used directly on a gel but this is comparatively insensitive, leads to many diffusion difficulties, and is not recommended for monoclonal antibodies.

10.5. Determination of antibody affinity

An approximate measure of antibody affinity is frequently required during screening so that high affinity antibodies may be selected. This can be achieved by screening hybridoma clones for specific antibody production and immunoglobulin production simultaneously. Supernatants which show strong specific antibody reaction with comparatively low amounts of immunoglobulin are more likely to have high affinity antibody.

Detailed measurements of monoclonal antibody affinity are in fact less complex to make than the equivalent measurements with conventional sera because of the lack of heterogeneity. The subject is covered in depth by Steward (1978). For soluble protein antigens, the equilibrium constant is most conveniently determined by radiolabelling the antigen with a γ label utilising a method which gives minimal structural damage such as iodogen (Pierce), lactoperoxidase, or methyl 3,5-diiodohydroxybenzimadate (Amersham) (see Johnson and Thorpe, 1982, for detailed discussion of labelling methodology). The radiolabelled antigen and monoclonal antibody are then reacted with each other over a wide range of antigen concentrations. The complex is then precipitated with 50 % ammonium sulphate or with a second anti-species antibody at optimal concentrations for precipitation and the proportion of antigen complexed to the fixed amount of antibody is determined at each antigen concentration.

Protocol 10.3

Determination of the affinity of a monoclonal antibody for a soluble protein antigen

(i) Radiolabel the antigen, preferably with ^{125}I utilising Iodogen, lactoperoxidase or methyl-3,5-diiodohydroxybenzimadate. The specific activity should ideally be close to 1 µCi/µg protein but lower specific activities will suffice. Check to see whether the antigen remains soluble in 50 % ammonium sulphate (see Note).

(ii) Grow the hybridoma clone to exhaustion to obtain large amounts of monoclonal antibody or grow the hybridoma in ascites fluid to produce the antibody.

(iii) In duplicate sets of 10 eppendorf tubes set up antigen dilutions over a concentration range of 10–200 µg antigen in 100 µl of phosphate-buffered saline. To each of one set of tubes add the monoclonal antibody in 50 µl of PBS at a concentration of 200–300 µg/ml. To each of the other set of tubes add tissue-culture supernatant or negative ascites fluid to serve as control. Incubate for 60 min at 4 °C.

(iv) To each tube add 150 µl of saturated ammonium sulphate and incubate at 4 °C for a further 30 min. Spin the tubes at 500 g for 5 min in a Beckman microfuge. Wash the precipitates twice with 50 % saturated ammonium sulphate and recentrifuge. Count the precipitates.

(v) For each antigen concentration estimate the total amount of antigen radioactivity and concentration in moles/1. Subtract the radioactivity in the precipitates from the control series of tubes from those in the test series to give a measure of the true antibody bound counts at each antigen concentration, and express this in moles/1. The concentration of free antigen is then the difference between total antigen concentration and bound antigen concentration.

Thus if the antigen was at a concentration of 10 µg/ml and has a molecular weight of 100 000 the total concentration will be 10^{-7} M. If this gives 200 000 counts/min and the bound antigen after subtraction of the control value gives 10 000 counts/min then the concentration of bound antigen is 5×10^{-9} M and the free antigen is 9.5×10^{-8} M. Obtain a series of results for bound (b) and free (c) antigen at all the concentrations employed.

(vi) The data may be plotted in two ways (Fig. 10.6). If the antibody concentration is not accurately known then according to the equation

$$1/b = 1/Kc(Ab_{\text{Tot}}) + 1/(Ab_{\text{Tot}})$$

a plot of $1/b$ against $1/c$ gives a measure of Ab_{Tot} which may be compared to the known concentration of monoclonal antibody. K, the equilibrium constant is the value of $1/c$ when exactly half the total antibody is bound to antigen.

An alternative approach is to plot according to the Sips equation (Steward, 1978).

$$\log (b/(Ab_{\text{Tot}} - b)) = a \log K + a \log c$$

Thus if $\log (b/(Ab_{\text{Tot}} - b))$ is plotted against $\log c$, $K = 1/c$ when the

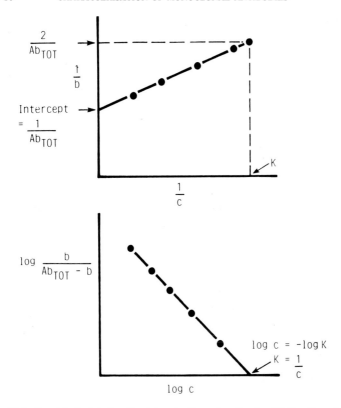

Fig. 10.6. Graphical plots for the determination of antibody affinity. Top, by the equation $1/b = 1/KcAb_{TOT} + 1/Ab_{TOT}$. Bottom, by the equation $\log(b/(Ab_{TOT} - b)) = a \log K + a \log c$. ($b$, bound antigen (moles/1); c, free antigen (moles/1).)

ordinate is zero. In this equation a is the 'heterogeneity' index which should be low for a monoclonal antibody.

Note. If the antigen is itself precipitated by ammonium sulphate then this method of separating bound and free antibody is unsuitable. The simplest alternative is to use a second anti-species antibody having previously determined the optimum precipitating conditions between this and the monoclonal antibody at the concentrations employed (Section 10.2.3). Such a method also removes doubts about the possible effects of the ammonium sulphate on the antibody–antigen interaction.

10.6. Karyotype analysis of hybridomas

Karyotyping is a skilled and complex technique and is probably best performed by genetics laboratories skilled in this particular task. It should be performed on all cell lines acquired from outside sources, particularly human ones, at the outset of any project. Cultures may readily be taken over by fast growing cell contaminants and there are many incidences of laboratories attempting to clone with cells which are not only of the wrong type but also of the wrong species. Karyotyping is also useful in the examination of the chromosome number of hybridomas and in the determination of which chromosomes are present in a cross-species fusion. A good light microscope is required.

The theoretical background to such techniques is based on the known effects of colchicine which inhibits microtubule polymerisation during mitosis. A consequence of this is that a high percentage of mitotic cells may be produced by treatment of the cells with colchicine. However, too much colchicine results in overcontracted chromosomes which are less readily identified and stained. There are a great variety of stains which may be used to identify human chromosomes in particular but the most generally employed one is Giemsa which gives very characteristic bands for each mammalian chromosome. The dye is not readily accessible to the chromosomes because of their protein coating which is more dense in the contracted state. Trypsin is therefore used to increase accessibility. However, too much trypsin releases the chromosomal DNA from its contracted condition and results in large diffusely stained chromosomes.

If only the number and general morphology of the chromosomes is required then the procedure given in Protocol 10.4 is comparatively simple. However, banding techniques are more complex. The Giemsa banding technique in Protocol 10.5 is dependent on the level of trypsinisation of the cells. Too much trypsin allows the chromosomes to expand so that identification becomes difficult. Too little gives minimal access to the stain. Banding techniques also require expertise in identification. The protocols below are given for lymphoblastoid and suspension cultures and differ from protocols used for fibro-blasts.

Protocol 10.4

Preparation of chromosome spreads

(i) Subculture 10 ml of cells at a density of $2-5 \times 10^5$/ml in 25-cm^2 flasks 24–48 h before karyotyping to make sure that they are in logarithmic growth. Prepare colchicine (Demecolcemid, Sigma) in 0.25-ml aliquots at 80 µg/ml in distilled water. This may be stored at $-20°$.

(ii) Add 25 µl of the stock colchicine solution for each 10 ml of cells in culture. Incubate for 90 min (a shorter time will produce less contracted chromosomes) and centrifuge for 5 min at 400 g in silicon-ised tubes. Pour off the supernatant and wash the cells in 0.14 M NaCl, 5 mM KCl, 0.5 mM EDTA, 0.2 % (w/v) phenol red, pH 7.4, recentrifuge and remove all but 2 ml of supernatant. Gently resus-pend the cells in this by tapping the tube. Add 10 ml 0.075 M KCl at 37°.

(iii) Incubate for 10 min at 37°. Centrifuge for 5 min at 400 g. Remove all but 0.2 ml of the supernatant and gently resuspend the cells by tapping the tube. Add 1 ml 3:1 methanol:acetic acid fixative (freshly prepared and cooled to 4°) slowly with shaking and then a further 9 ml. Seal the tube and place at 4° for at least 30 min and several hours if this is more suitable.

(iv) Centrifuge for 5 min at 400 g, resuspend in 10 ml fresh fixative and recentrifuge. Resuspend in 1 ml fresh fixative.

(v) Using a siliconised Pasteur pipette held close to the ear, drop the cell suspension onto a wet glass slide held at arm's length. Dry the slide and examine at low magnification.

Note. If there are problems due to cell clumping then the 10-min incubation in 0.075 M KCl in step (ii) may be replaced by the addition of 6 drops of fixative followed by immediate centrifugation. This may reduce the quality of the spreads.

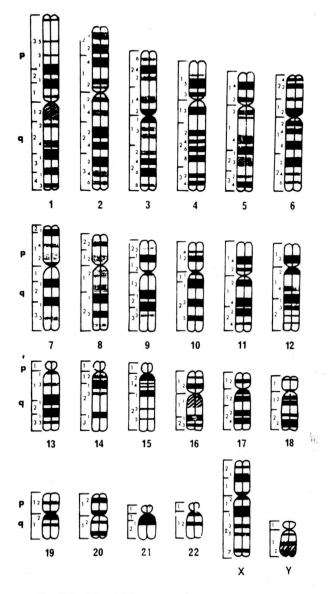

Fig. 10.7. G-banded karyotype of normal human cells.

Protocol 10.5

Giemsa staining of chromosome spreads

(i) Prepare a solution of trypsin (Difco-Bacto Code 0153-59) in 10 ml normal (0.9 %) saline. Aliquot in 0.5-ml portions and store at −20°. Use aliquots as required and do not refreeze. After thawing dilute samples around the range of 0.4 ml trypsin to 25 ml normal saline.

(ii) Place the dried slide in a slide rack in a covered container with 2 × SSC (0.3 M NaCl, 0.03 M Na citrate pH 7). Incubate at 60° for 2 h. Remove the slide rack to containers with firstly 0.15 M NaCl and secondly distilled water to rinse.

(iii) Dehydrate the slides by moving the slide rack sequentially for 2-min intervals to 50%, then 70%, 90%, 95%, and 100% ethanol and air dry.

(iv) Place a trial slide in the diluted trypsin solution for 70–80 sec and rinse immediately in normal saline. Stain the slide in a fresh solution containing 4 parts BDH pH 6.8 buffer (BDH Gurr code 33199) and one part Leishman's stain (0.15 g Leishman's powder in 100 ml methanol stirred cold for 2 h and filtered before use) for 3.5 min and rinse in pH 6.8 buffer immediately. Dry the slide on a hot or warm plate.

(v) Examine the slide under the microscope. If the chromosomes show little stain in the bands then increase the time in trypsin for a few seconds. If they appear bloated and diffuse then decrease it. If the banding is visible but of unsuitable intensity and the chromosome morphology is normal, then alter the time in the stain accordingly. It is likely that the two variables (trypsin time and stain time) may have to be altered several times to obtain an ideal identification.

(vi) Photograph the slide, cut out and pair the photographs of the individual chromosomes and compare with the normal human karyotype (Fig. 10.7).

.Animal handling techniques

A.1.1. Introduction

Detailed information on animal handling techniques may be found in texts such as Williams and Chase (1967) and Herbert (1973). However, most of the procedures relevant to rodent hybridoma production are described below.

A.1.2. Requirement for Home Office Licence

In the U.K., any laboratory worker needs to be licensed by the Home Office to carry out procedures which might cause pain to laboratory animals. The licence, under the Cruelty to Animals Act (1876), exempts the experimenter from prosecution for cruelty to animals when carrying out the particular procedures for which he is licensed. Before undertaking experimental work with animals, investigators should write to The Home Office, Queen Anne's Gate, London SW1H 9AT with an enquiry concerning a licence to cover them for the work.

A.1.3. Handling

A.1.3.1. Identification

Individual animals in the same cage will often need to be identified for repeated immunizations or other procedures. The most satisfacto-

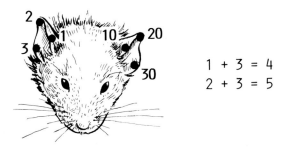

$$1 + 3 = 4$$
$$2 + 3 = 5$$

Fig. A.1.1. A system of earclips for animal identification.

ry permanent methods for identifying mice and rats are by ear clips, or by dyeing the fur. The system of ear clips illustrated in Figure A.1.1 uses three positions on each ear.

Fur dyes in use include picric acid and gentian violet. Aqueous solutions of the dyes should be diluted with alcohol to decrease the

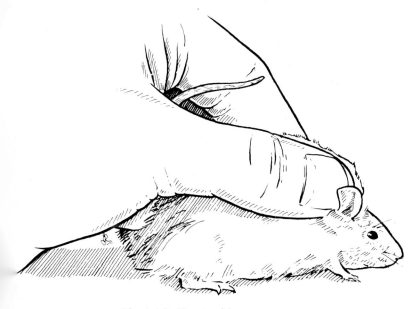

Fig. A.1.2. How to pick up a mouse.

drying time. Six positions are convenient to use, shoulder, flank, and rump, on the right and left sides. The dyes are best applied with cotton-tipped applicators, which should be inserted under the outer fur, and rolled so as to dye in the underfur.

A.1.3.2. Restraint

Mice should be picked up by the tail, near the base, and placed on a grid. When the tail is pulled gently, the animal holds on to the grid with its feet, and it can then be picked up by grasping the loose skin over the shoulders with the thumb and forefinger, while the tail is held with the little finger (Fig. A.1.2). For intravenous injection or for bleeding from the tail, a restraint consisting of a wire mesh tube, closed at one end, is used (Fig. A.1.3). When the mouse's head is put into the tube, it will enter it, and it can then be confined there by a bung with a notch in one side through which the tail protrudes.

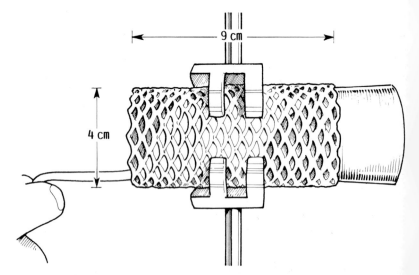

Fig. A.1.3. Tube restraint for mouse. Most mice will hold on to the mesh in the tubing with their claws. An uncooperative animal is restrained with a grooved bung in the rear end of the tube so that only the tail is visible.

A.1.3.3. Anaesthesia

For anaesthetising animals for short periods of time, ether is usually satisfactory. The ether jar should be arranged with a grid over the cotton wool soaked in ether, so that the animal only breathes the fumes, but does not come in contact with the ether, which will irritate the skin. The animal is sufficiently anaesthetised when the breathing is regular and slow, and when it does not twitch if a foot is gently pinched. Additional ether may be administered during the course of an operation by placing a small beaker with ether-soaked cotton wool in the bottom, over the animal's head.

For anaesthetising mice for longer periods of time, intraperitoneal injection of a barbiturate, such as Sagatal (May and Baker) is used. It should be diluted in ethanol and water (Sagatal:ethanol:distilled water, 1:1:10), and injected at a dose of approximately 0.01 ml per g body weight. There are genetic (strain) differences in susceptibility to barbiturate anaesthetics.

A.1.3.4. Euthanasia

Animals may be quickly killed with CO_2 either from a cylinder or in the form of frozen pellets. The vapour is heavy, so the animal should be at the bottom of the container into which the gas is introduced.

A.1.4. Immunization

A.1.4.1. Intraperitoneal

Needle size: 23G or 25G.
Maximum amount to be injected: up to 2 ml in large mouse, up to 1 ml in smaller strains.
The mouse is held by grasping the loose skin over the shoulders with the thumb and forefinger, and holding the base of the tail with the little finger, belly upwards. The needle is inserted to a depth of

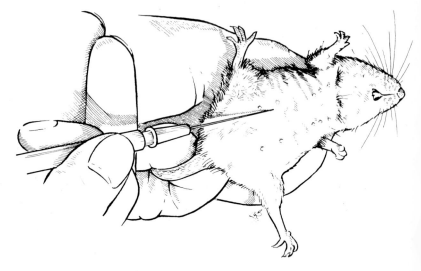

Fig. A.1.4. Intraperitoneal injection.

approximately 5 mm, to one side of the midline, between the lower two nipples (Fig. A.1.4). Injections at the midline may enter the urinary bladder, and an injection too high in the peritoneal cavity may damage liver or spleen. The inoculum should be injected slowly, and there should be a brief pause before the needle is withdrawn, to allow the inoculum to disseminate. If there is a swelling at the injection site, the injection has been subcutaneous, not intraperitoneal.

A.1.4.2. Subcutaneous

Needle size: 23G or 25G.
Maximum amount: 0.2 ml.

The mouse is placed on a grid, and the loose skin and tail held as before. The animal should be left on the grid and gently held down by the backs of the third and fourth fingers of the left hand. The needle is inserted through the skin at the back of the neck, and pointing posteriorly, so that the point is below the fingers holding the skin. The point should be moved in a short arc to check that it moves freely between skin and body. The inoculum is injected, and the fingers should then be moved to grasp the site of needle penetration as the needle is withdrawn, to prevent loss of the inoculum through the hole in the skin.

A.1.4.3. Intravenous

Needle size: 25G or 26G.
Maximum amount: 0.2 ml.

Intravenous injections in mice are neither quick nor easy, and practice is needed before the necessary skill can be acquired. It should be attempted first on albino mice, as their veins are easier to see. Some

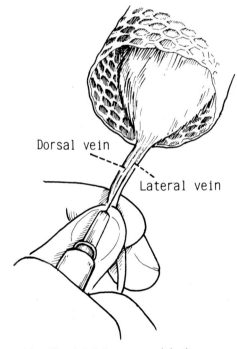

Dorsal vein

Lateral vein

Fig. A.1.5. Intravenous injection.

people prefer using an all-glass syringe, because the plunger moves more easily than in a plastic syringe. Great care should be taken that all air bubbles are expelled from the syringe, hub, and needle before injection. The mouse should be restrained in a wire mesh tube with the tail protruding, as described above. Vasodilation should be induced either by warming the mouse with a desk lamp, or by warming the tail with cotton wool dipped in warm water. It is best to use the lateral tail veins, and to make the first injection distally, as a second attempt can then be made in a more proximal position. The mouse's tail should be held over the forefinger of the left hand, and the needle inserted into the vein on the straight part of the tail just over the finger (Fig. A.1.5). As the inoculum is injected, there should be no resistance and the vein should be seen to clear. If there is resistance as the plunger is pushed, and if the tail blanches, the injection has been subcutaneous.

A.1.4.4. Intramuscular

Needle size: 25G.
Maximum amount: 0.05 ml.

An assistant is required to hold the mouse while the experimenter extends the hind leg and makes the injection into the thigh muscle above the femur. The needle should approach from behind the animal and be pointed along the femur toward the body.

A.1.4.5. Intradermal

Needle size: 25G or 26G.
Maximum amount: 0.05 ml.

The skin should be shaved over a site on the back of the mouse. A fold of skin is pinched up between thumb and forefinger, and the needle inserted just below the surface of the skin, along the fold. The needle should be visible below the surface of the skin. When the inoculum is injected, the skin should blanche, and a pea-like swelling should appear just below the surface.

A.1.4.6. Footpad

Needle size: 25G or 26G.
Maximum amount: 0.025 ml.

Because of the discomfort to the animal, this site should only be used if the draining lymph node is required. Only a hind foot should be used, as mice manipulate food with the forepaws. An assistant is needed to hold the mouse, while the experimenter extends the hind leg and injects the inoculum just under the surface of the footpad.

A.1.4.7. Oral

Maximum amount: 2 ml.

Two kinds of fitting are used for oral dosing of mice. One is a cannula with a Luer fitting and a rounded metal end (Fig. A.1.6). The other apparatus is made by cleanly cutting and fire-polishing a short piece of narrow polythene tubing and then fitting it over a 19G or 21G needle. The mouse should be held by an assistant with its head back so that the throat and oesophagus are lined up as straight as possible. The cannula is slid gently down the throat as far as the stomach. If resistance is encountered before the cannula has penetrated as far as the stomach, the cannula may have entered the trachea. The cannula should then be withdrawn, and a second attempt made.

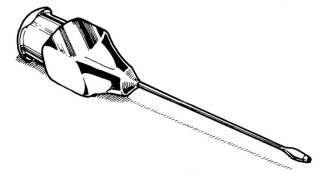

Fig. A.1.6. Fitting for oral immunisation of mice.

A.1.5. Serum collection

A.1.5.1. Bleeding from the tail

Two methods may be used to obtain blood from the tail of a mouse. Firstly, a sharp scalpel or razor blade may be used to cut a small piece off the end of the tail, and the drops of blood can be collected with a capillary tube or a pasteur pipette. When sufficient blood has been collected (not more than 100 µl if the animal is to be bled repeatedly) the bleeding should be stopped by pressure of the fingers.

Alternatively, a sharp scalpel blade may be used to make a slanting cut in one of the lateral tail veins, and the blood collected and the bleeding stopped as before (Fig. A.1.7).

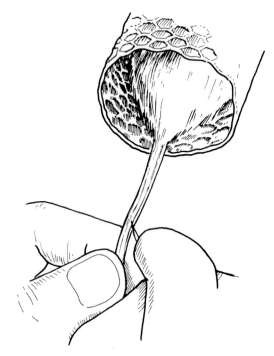

Fig. A.1.7. Bleeding from the lateral tail vein.

A.1.5.2. Serum separation

The blood should be collected into narrow glass or plastic tubes (e.g. Sarstedt 0.4 ml polythene tubes). If a large volume of blood has been collected, e.g. at exsanguination, a wooden toothpick may be put in the tube. The clot forms around the toothpick and is easily removed by taking the toothpick out of the tube. However, the use of a toothpick is not advisable with small volumes of blood (50–100 µl). Mouse blood is rather subject to haemolysis, so the clot should be allowed to form at room temperature (rather than at 37°) for 30–40 min. The clot should then be detached from the side of the tube by flicking the tube vigorously, and the tube left at 4° overnight to allow the clot to retract. The serum may then be removed with a capillary tube, using mouth suction through a narrow polythene tube.

A.1.6. Removal of tissues at sacrifice

A.1.6.1. Exsanguination

A.1.6.1.1. Cardiac puncture   This method is often used if the sterile removal of the spleen is to follow the collection of blood. The mouse is killed with CO_2 and immediately after breathing has stopped the thoracic cavity is carefully opened by cutting the ribs to one side of the sternum. A 21G needle is inserted into the right ventricle and blood is slowly withdrawn from the heart, which is still beating.

A.1.6.1.2. Inferior vena cava   This is the method of choice when the maximum amount of blood is required. As soon as breathing has stopped the peritoneal cavity is opened and the gut is reflected. A 21G needle is inserted just proximal to the kidneys into the inferior vena cava (arrowed in Fig. A.1.8).

The blood is drawn slowly into the syringe, allowing time for the blood to drain into the vein, and making sure that the bevel of the needle is not blocked against the vein wall.

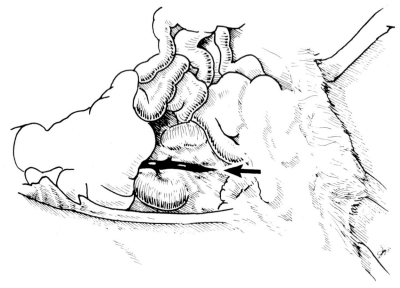

Fig. A.1.8. Inferior vena cava.

A.1.6.2. Tissues containing immune cells

A.1.6.2.1. Spleen   If the cells are needed for culture, the tissues must be sterilely removed from the animal. Two pairs of forceps and two scissors are required. They should be clean, dipped in 70% alcohol, and flamed before use. The mouse should be killed with CO_2, placed on its back for dissection, and soaked with 70% alcohol. The first set of scissors and forceps should be used to cut and reflect the skin over the abdomen. The second set of scissors and forceps should then be used to make a cut in the peritoneal wall on the mouse's left side. The spleen lies on the left side (from the mouse's point of view) of the peritoneal cavity, just below the stomach (Fig. A.1.9). The veins and connective tissue by which it is attached all lie on the side of the organ toward the peritoneal cavity.

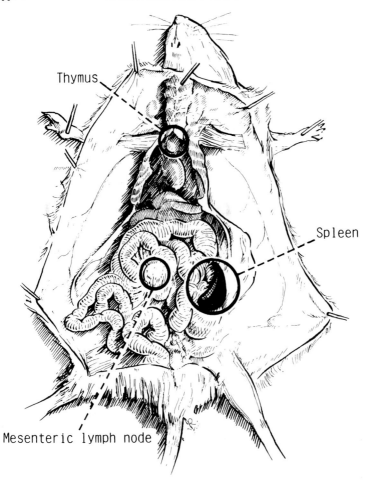

Fig. A.1.9. Spleen, thymus and mesenteric lymph nodes.

A.1.6.2.2. Lymph nodes   For the sterile removal of lymph nodes the mouse should be treated as for the removal of the spleen. The lymph nodes yield only small numbers of cells, and several may be required to get a sufficient cell yield. They do yield lymphocytes uncontaminated by red blood cells. In the mouse, the cervical, brachi-

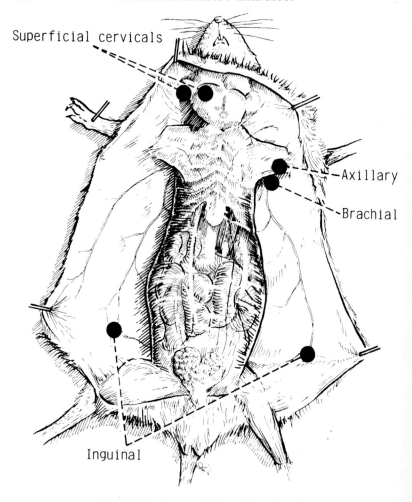

Fig. A.1.10. Some easily located lymph nodes.

al, axillary, and inguinal nodes are easily found, and drain different areas of the body (Fig. A.1.10). The mesenteric node, which is attached to the large intestine, is a bigger node (Fig. A.1.9). It drains the gut wall, but not antigen injected intraperitoneally.

A.1.6.2.3. Thymus   The thymus is a bilobed, soft tissue which is ventral, and just anterior, to the heart (Fig. A.1.9). It is reached by first reflecting the skin and muscle layer over the sternum. The ribs are then cut at either side of the sternum, along most of its length. The thymus is a greyish mass at the top of the thoracic cavity. It is attached at its anterior aspect. If a suspension of pure thymocytes is required, the two parathymic lymph nodes must be removed before teasing the tissue to obtain cells.

A.1.6.2.4. Peritoneal cells   The cells which can be washed from the peritoneal cavity consist of a mixture of macrophages (activated or normal), lymphocytes, polymorphonuclear cells, mast cells and eosinophils. The proportions of these types of cells varies with the health of the animal and its experimental treatment. The use of inducing agents alters the proportion and state of the cell types present and the timing of peritoneal lavage after the use of inducing agents is important if particular cell types are required. To obtain peritoneal

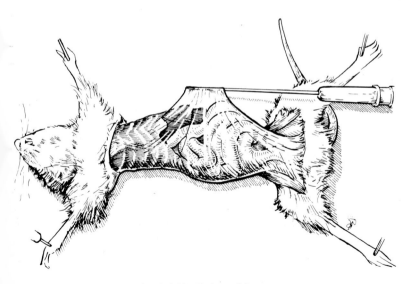

Fig. A.1.11. Peritoneal lavage.

cells, the dead mouse should be placed on its back on a dissecting board or tray and soaked in 70% alcohol, as before. A cut should be made in the abdominal skin and the skin pulled away with the fingers towards the animal's head and tail, so that the whole peritoneal wall is exposed. Approximately 2–3 ml of medium should be injected at the midline with a 25G needle. The mouse carcase is then massaged to disperse the medium throughout the peritoneal cavity. A 21G needle is then inserted through the peritoneal wall, pointing anteriorly, and with the point lying beside the spleen. The needle is gently pulled to the side, so that a pocket of fluid forms beside the spleen, and the fluid is slowly drawn into the syringe, allowing time for more fluid to seep into the pocket, and avoiding the needle being clogged by the nearby fat (Fig. A.1.11).

A.1.7. Ascites fluid

A.1.7.1. Induction

Suspensions of cells may be grown in ascites fluids in mice. The mouse to be used should be 'primed' by the intraperitoneal injection of 0.5 ml Pristane (2,6,10,14-tetramethyl pentadecane, Aldrich). 4–10 days after priming, 1.5×10^6 cells are injected intraperitoneally (Section 9.3).

The time taken for the ascitic fluid to develop is very variable, from 5 to 11 days, being average. The fluid should be drained when the mouse has swollen to approximately the proportions of a pregnant female near term.

A.1.7.2. Tapping of fluid

Two methods may be used. For either method the mouse must be lightly anaesthetized with ether. The first method is to hold the anaesthetized mouse over a beaker, use a 21G needle to make a hole in the abdominal skin and peritoneal wall, and allow the ascitic fluid to drip through the hole and into the beaker. Sterile collection of the ascitic fluid may alternatively be done by a method similar to that used for peritoneal lavage. The anaesthetized mouse is placed on its back, and a 21G needle is inserted into the peritoneum at the animal's left side, with the needle pointing anteriorly and with the point to one side of the spleen. The fluid is then drawn slowly into the syringe.

Addresses of suppliers and manufacturers

Aldrich Chemical Company
New Road, Gillingham
Dorset SP8 4BR
U.K.

Amersham International, Alpha Laboratories Ltd.
White Lion Road, Amersham
Bucks HP7 9LL
U.K.

Amicon Ltd.
Upper Mill, Stonehouse, Gloucestershire
GL10 2BJ
U.K.

Amicon Corporation
21 Hartwell Ave, Lexington
MA 02173
U.S.A.

BDH Chemicals Ltd.
Poole, Dorset
U.K.

Beckman-RIIC Ltd.
Sands Industrial Estate
High Wycombe, Bucks, U.K.
Irvine, CA 92713
U.S.A.

Becton Dickinson UK Ltd.
Between Towns Road, Cowley, Oxford
OX4 3LY
U.K.

Becton Dickinson
Oxnrd, CA 93030
U.S.A.

Bio-Rad Laboratories
Caxton Way, Watford, Herts
WD1 8RP, U.K. 2200
Wright Avenue, Richmond, CA 94804
U.S.A.

Boehringer-Mannheim
Bell Lane, Lewes, Sussex
BN7 1LG
U.K.

Boehringer-Mannheim
GmbH, Biochimica
D-6800 Mannheim 31
West-Germany.

Celltech Ltd.
244–250 Bath Rd
Slough SLI Bucks
U.K.

Costar
205 Broadway, Cambridge, MA 02139
U.S.A.
U.K. Suppliers, Northumbria Biologicals
Ltd.
Cramlington, Northumbria NE23 9HL,
U.K.

Cryotech (Cryoson)
Frogmore Lane, Stanford in the Vale
Oxon SN7 8LG, U.K.

Difco
Central Ave., West Mosely
Surrey KT 0SE U.K.
P.O. Box 1058A, Detroit, ML 48232
U.S.A.

Dynatech Laboratories Ltd.
Billinghurst, Sussex RH14 9SJ, U.K.
900 Slaters Lane, Alexandria, VA 22314
U.S.A.

Eppendorf, Gerateban, Netheler and Hinz
P.O. Box 630324, 2000, Hamburg 63,
West-Germany
U.K. Suppliers Anderman and Co.
Central Ave., E. Molesey
Surrey KT8 OQZ
U.K.

Falcon Plastics
see Becton Dickinson.

Flow Laboratories
P.O. Box 17, Irvine, Ayrshire KA12 8NB
U.K.
7655 Old Springhouse Road
McLean, VA 22102, U.S.A.

Gallenkamp and Co. Ltd
P.O. Box 290, Christopher St.
London EC2P 2ER, U.K.

Gilson France S.A.
B.P. No. 45-95400, Villiers le Bel, France
U.K. Suppliers Anachem Ltd.
15 Power Court, Luton, Beds LU2 7QE
U.K.

Gibco Ltd.
Trident House, Renfrew Road, Paisley
PA3 4EF
U.K.

Hoechst, U.K. Ltd.
Hoechst   House,   Salisbury   Road,
Hounslow

Middlesex TW4 6JH
U.K.

Hopkin and Williams
Freshwater Road, Chadwell Heath, Essex
U.K.

Kodak Ltd.
Station Road
Hemel Hampstead, HP1 1JU
U.K.

L.K.B. Instruments Ltd.
232, Addington Road
S. Croydon CR2 8YD, U.K.
L.K.B. Productor AB
Box 305 S-161 26 Bromma
Sweden.

Miles Laboratories Ltd.
P.O. Box 37, Stoke Poges
Slough, SL2 4LY, U.K.
Elkhart, IN 46515
U.S.A.

Millipore Corporation
Harrow, Middlesex, HA1 2HY, U.K
Bradford, MA 01730
U.S.A.

New England Nuclear
2 New Rd., Southampton SO2 OAA,
U.K.
NEN Corporation, Boston, MA
U.S.A.

Nunc, see Gibco.

Nordic Immunological Labs.
2, St. Peters Rd., Maidenhead
Berks SL6 7QU, U.K.
P.O. Box 22, Tilburg
The Netherlands.

OLAC (1976) Ltd.
Shaw's Farm, Blackthorn
Bicester OX6 OTP
U.K.

Olympus, see Gallenkamp.

Pharmacia (G.B.) Ltd.
Prince Regent Rd., Hounslow
Middlesex TW3 1NE, U.K.
Pharmacia AB, Box 175, S-75104 Uppsala
Sweden.

Pierce and Warriner U.K.
Chester, Cheshire CH1 4EF, U.K.
Pierce Chem Co., Box 117, Rockford
IL 61105, U.S.A.

Schleicher and Schull
Postfach 4, D-3354 Dassel, W. Germany
Anderman and Co., Central Ave
East Molesley, Surrey KT8 OQZ, U.K.
Keene, NH 03431
U.S.A.

Sera-Lab Ltd.
Crawley, Down, Sussex
U.K.

Shandon
Broad St., Sewickley
PA 15143
U.S.A.

Sigma Chem. Co. Ltd.
Fancy Rd., Poole
Dorset BH17 7NH, U.K.
Sigma Chemical Co., P.O. Box 14508
St. Louis, MO 63178
U.S.A.

Sterilin Ltd.
Teddington, Middlesex TW11 8QZ
U.K.

Techne, Duxford
Cambridge, CB2 4PZ, U.K.
Brunswick Pike, Princeton, NJ
U.S.A.

Whatman Chem. Ltd.
Springfield, Maidenstone
Kent ME14 2LE, U.K.
9 Bridewell Place, Cliften, NJ 07014
U.S.A.

Note. **Gibco** has recently merged with **BRL** to form *Life Technologies* and material may be marketed under this name in future.

Protocols for polyacrylamide gel electrophoresis (PAGE)

A.3.1. Introduction

Whole volumes in this series have been written on the electrophoretic separation of proteins (e.g. Righetti, 1983). In addition, standard immunological or biochemical methods textbooks give much greater detail than can be supplied here (see for example Hames and Rickwood, 1981, or Johnson and Thorpe, 1982). The information given below relates to the electrophoretic techniques most commonly employed in hybridoma technology.

Polyacrylamide gel analysis is widely used in the characterisation of both a monoclonal antibody and its antigen. It is used in particular for determination of the class of secreted antibody (Section 10.2.3), for proof of monoclonality (Section 10.3) and for immunoblotting (Section 10.4.4). Only slab gels are suitable for most of these procedures.

A.3.2. Slab gel apparatus

Slab gels are poured into two glass plates typically 18 cm × 13 cm clamped vertically together with spacers holding the plates apart. Spacers are made of plexiglas and are of thickness 1–5 mm. Thin gels are generally more suitable for autoradiographic procedures. Thicker gels hold more protein and may be more suitable for immunoblotting of minor proteins. One of the glass plates has a groove 2 cm deep and approximately 14 cm long on one of the long (18 cm) sides. When the gel is poured a 'comb' made of plexiglas of the same thickness as the spacers is inserted into this groove while the gel sets. The comb is removed before sample application into the slots it creates in the gel. The number of teeth in the comb is a matter of choice relating to the number of samples to be run, their volume, and the expertise of the operator.

The gel is poured in liquid form and will obviously leak out the bottom of such an apparatus unless great care is taken. Leakage can be stopped by greasing the spacers with petroleum jelly and using a third spacer along the bottom of the gel and sealing the possible leakage points with a small amount of fast setting 1.5% agar at the edges. It is also effectively stopped by running a length of 2 mm diameter flexible silicone tubing round the edge of the plates outside the spacers. A third method involves the use of thin, plastic backed sticky tape around the outside of the outside of the glass plates. The two plates are firmly clamped together with foldback office clips. Commercial apparatus of this type is readily obtained (e.g. Bio-Rad or Shandon).

A.3.3. SDS–PAGE (sodium dodecyl sulphate–polyacrylamide gel electrophoresis)

SDS–PAGE separates proteins on the basis of size. The SDS denatures the proteins to give a uniform tertiary structure and binds to most proteins to the same extent (exceptions are highly charged proteins such as histones, and glycoproteins). The PAGE has a molecular sieving effect so that small proteins move more readily through the gel. Gel concentrations are usually in the region of 10%. Lower percentages are used for large proteins and higher percentages for small proteins. Gels of 5% polyacrylamide and below are extremely difficult to handle.

The gel mould is prepared and the ingredients for the main gel are made up according to the information in Table A.3.1. Acrylamide and bis-acrylamide are neurotoxins and should be handled with

TABLE A.3.1
Composition of SDS–polyacrylamide gels (SDS–PAGE) (50 ml)

	5%	7.5%	10%	12.5%
Stock acrylamide solution (48.75% w/v acrylamide 1.25% w/v N,N'-methylene bisacrylamide)	5	7.5	10	12.5
1.5 M Tris–HCl, pH 8.7	12.5	12.5	12.5	12.5
Water	30.8	28.3	25.8	23.3
10% (w/v) SDS	0.5	0.5	0.5	0.5
1% (w/v) ammonium persulphate (fresh)	1.2	1.2	1.2	1.2
TEMED (N,N,N',N'-tetramethyl-ethylamine diamine)	0.02	0.02	0.02	0.02

gloves. The gel is degassed *before* the addition of SDS, ammonium persulphate and TEMED (Table A.3.1). The TEMED catalyses the polymerisation and consequently its concentration affects the speed with which the gel sets. Too high a concentration leads to the gel setting before it is properly poured and too low to very slow setting. The ammonium persulphate must be made up *immediately* before use. The gel is poured into the mould to 3–4 cm from the top, immediately overlayed with water saturated butanol and allowed to set. In most laboratories this is performed by leaving the gel at room temperature but the gel may also be set in a 37° water bath to accelerate the polymerisation.

When the main gel has polymerised the butanol is removed and the top of the gel is gently rinsed with the buffer to be used for the stacking gel. The stacking gel is then prepared according to Table A.3.2. A 5% stacking gel is generally used as a 3% one is hard to handle but 3% stacking gels are necessary where the main gel is 5% or lower. The stacking gel is then poured and the comb is inserted so that the teeth are 0.5–1 cm above the main gel. The stacking gel should polymerise in 30 min. The side spacers remain in place but the bottom spacer or

TABLE A.3.2
Composition of stacking gel (10 ml) for SDS–PAGE

	3%	5%
Stock acrylamide solution (48.75% acrylamide, 1.25% N,N'-methylene bisacrylamide)	0.6	1.0
1 M Tris–HCl, pH 6.8	1.25	1.25
Water	7.5	7.1
10% (w/v) SDS	0.1	0.1
1% (w/v) ammonium persulphate (fresh)	0.5	0.5
TEMED (N,N,N',N'-tetramethyl-ethylamine diamine)	0.01	0.01

sticky tape or silicone tubing is then removed and the gel is clamped vertically to the electrophoresis apparatus with the bottom of the comb notch level with the lip of the top electrophoresis chamber. Vaseline or petroleum jelly are generally employed to seal the two. Both chambers are filled with the electrophoresis buffer (0.025 M Tris, 0.192 M glycine, 0.1% (w/v) SDS pH 8.3) and the comb is then carefully removed.

The samples are prepared by mixing with an equal volume of 2 × sample buffer (0.125 M Tris–HCl pH 6.8, 5% (w/v) SDS, 10% (v/v) 2-mercaptoethanol, 20% (v/v) glycerol, and 0.005% bromophenol blue pH 6.8) and heating in a boiling water bath for 2 min. Standard proteins of known molecular weight are also prepared for running in a separate track of the gel. The samples are loaded carefully with an eppendorf pipette or Hamilton syringe. The exact volume depends on the size of the teeth of the comb but the dye detection system should detect less than 1 µg of protein band. Radioactive detection systems are obviously very much more sensitive.

The electrodes are connected so that the sample runs down the gel towards the anode and the gel is run at a constant current of 20–30 mA for the size of slab described. The progress may be monitored by the bromophenol blue. At the end of the electrophoresis, the gel is carefully removed and either used for Western blotting (Section 10.4.4) or put into a large container with the staining solution (0.25% Coumassie brilliant blue in methanol:acetic acid:distilled water, 5:1:5) which is more effective if prewarmed to 37° and shaken slowly for 45 − 60 min. It is destained in methanol:acetic acid:distilled water 5:1:5 with several changes until the bands become visible above the background. Again, the process is more efficient if the stain is warm.

A.3.4. Urea polyacrylamide gel electrophoresis

This process is one which solubilises most proteins but is less extreme than SDS–polyacrylamide gel electrophoresis. It is therefore sometimes more suitable for Western blotting of antigens which do not readily renature from SDS solutions. It does not yield information on the molecular weight of the antigen. Acid urea gels were commonly used in the 1970s for the dectection of basic proteins which blot well (Towbin et al., 1979). Acid urea gels are prepared and run in 0.1 M formate or citrate buffer pH 4.5–5.5. The procedures are similar to the alkaline ones described below.

The sample is usually prepared in 8 M urea containing 2% (w/v) dithiothreitol. The stock gel solution is 5.6% (w/v) acrylamide, 0.28% (w/v) N,N'-methylene bisacrylamide, 6 M urea, 0.3 M Tris–HCl pH 8.8. This is degassed. To a 50-ml aliquot, 1 ml of 1.5% ammonium sulphate is added and then 0.02 ml TEMED. The gel is immediately poured into the vertical apparatus and allowed to set with the comb in place. Sample application is as in Section A.3.3. The electrode buffer is 0.05 M sodium borate pH 9.2.

A.3.5. Isoelectric focussing of immunoglobulins

This technique has its main application in hybridoma technology in the demonstration of antibody homogeneity. It is, however, not suitable for IgM molecules if polyacrylamide is used and agarose gels are generally employed in these cases (Rosen et al., 1979). The type of agarose employed is critical and special material is marketed by Pharmacia and LKB for this purpose.

Isoelectric focussing equipment may be obtained at considerable cost from most commercial suppliers (Pharmacia, LKB). There is a considerable size variation to the available plates and a small gel is most easily run as these gels are usually at a low percentage of acrylamide. One plate is removed after the gel has been poured and consequently this is usually siliconised prior to the pouring of the gel. The other plate on which the gel is run is frequently coated with a protein solution such as chromium-hardened gelatin to avoid tearing and distortion of the gel. Alternatively, the polyacrylamide may be covalently attached to specially coated plates (Nicolotti et al., 1980). The gel is poured vertically and can be run vertically but it is more commonly run in a flatbed electrophoresis tank. Spacers are usually 10 mm thickness because of gel fragility but thinner gels may be used.

The acrylamide gel solution is 5% (w/v) acrylamide and 0.25% (w/v) N,N'-methylene bisacrylamide together with the stock ampholines. For antibody solutions they usually also contain 3 M urea which is only necessary if the sample has been reduced. The stock ampholines are purchased at 40% and used at 2%. Ampholines cover a variety of pH ranges and it is usually best to mix two sets covering the pH range 5–7 and 7–9 each at a concentration of 2%. Polymerisation is by the addition of riboflavin (0.1 mg/ml) and TEMED (30 µl/100 ml of solution) just before the gel is poured followed by fluorescent illumination of the gel for 3–4 h. A sample comb may be used if a vertical gel is to be run. However, it is more usual to remove the siliconised plate gently from the top of the polymerised gel and lay the gel on the bottom plate on a flatbed electrophoresis tank.

Samples are usually reduced to allow for resolution of both light

and heavy chain and are prepared in 6 M urea, 5% (v/v) β-mercapto-
ethanol, 0.1 M phosphate buffer pH 8. They are warmed to 37° for
30 min and then applied directly to 0.5 cm × 3 cm strips of Whatman
3mm filter paper for flatbed electrophoresis. The strips are placed on
the gel about 1 cm from the anode.

The anode buffer is 5% phosphoric acid and the cathode one 5%
ethylenediamine. Close contact between the gel and the electrodes is
helpful and this may be performed by placing the gel directly onto
graphite electrodes with the sample on the anodic side but not
touching the anode. Alternatively, the electrodes may be placed on
the gel. If the plate on which the gel lies is not coated with gelatin to
hold the gel the latter process is essential. Paper wicks (Whatman
3mm) are used to form contacts between the anodic and cathodic
buffers and the gel surface. Focussing is approached gradually starting at a current of 5 mA/plate, increasing the voltage stepwise over
a period of 2 h. The plate is then focussed overnight at 450 V for a
20-cm gel. In the morning the voltage may be further increased to 600
V for a 20-cm gel for another hour.

The apparatus is then switched off and the pH gradient is measured
with a flat membrane electrode. The gel is then fixed with 3.5% (w/v)
sulphosalicylic acid, 11.5% (w/v) trichloroacetic acid and autoradiographed and/or stained and destained as in Section A.3.3.

A.3.6. Autoradiography or fluorography of gels

In autoradiography the direct emission from the isotope is measured.
In fluorography the energy is converted into light which is more
efficient in exposing X-ray film. Fluorography is essential for weak
β-emitting isotopes.

For autoradiography the gel is dried down by vacuum of a special
apparatus (Pharmacia, Bio-Rad). The gel is placed on a rubber sheet
and overlayed with Whatman 3mm filter paper, a second perforated
rubber sheet and a nylon sinter. The fluid is then drawn out by a
vacuum pump.

The dried gel is then placed (in the dark) onto a sheet of Kodak X-Omat S film and the two are clamped between glass plates and secured in several layers of black plastic. Intensifying screens are generally used for high-energy isotopes. Exposure is for 2 days at $-70°$ to prolong the half life of the silver atoms. The gel can be exposed to fresh film for a longer or shorter time period if this is unsuitable.

In fluorography, the gel is photographed after destaining since the stain will be removed by the fluorography. It is then soaked in pure dimethyl sulphoxide (DMSO) for 1 h and then incubated in 17% 2,5-diphenyloxazole (PPO) in DMSO for a further 4 h in the dark. It is washed with water and dried as for autoradiography. Exposure is with a light sensitive film such as Fuji RX and is for a shorter time than that required for autoradiography but also at $-70°$.

References

ABRAMS, P.G., KNOST, J.A., CLARKE, G., WILBURN, S. and OLDHAM, R.K. (1983) J. Immunol. *131*, 1201.

ADAMS, R.L.P. (1980) Cell Culture for Biochemists. Laboratory Techniques in Biochemistry and Molecular Biology, Eds. Work, T.S., and Burdon, R.H., Elsevier.

AHKONG, Q.F., FISHER, D., TAMPION, W. and LUCY, J.A. (1973) Biochem. J. *136*, 147.

AK-KAISSI, E. and MOSTRATOS, A. (1983) J. Immunol. Meth. *58*, 127.

ANDERSSON, J., COUTHINO, A. and MELCHERS, F. (1979) J. Exp. Med. *149*, 553.

ALBERTINI, A. and EKINS, R. (Eds.) (1981) Monoclonal Antibodies and Developments in Immunoassay, Elsevier.

ALBERTINI, R.J. and DEMARS, R. (1973) Mutation Res. *18*, 199.

ARNOLD, B., BATTYE, F.L. and MILLER, J.F.A.P. (1979) J. Immunol. Meth. *29*, 353.

ASHALL, F., BRAMWELL, M.E. and HARRIS, H. (1982) Lancet, 3rd July.

ASTALDI, G.C.B., JANSSEN, M.C., LANSDORP, P., WILLEMS, C., ZEIJLMAKER, W.P. and OOSTERHOF, F. (1980) J. Immunol. *125*, 1411.

ASTALDI, G.C.B., WRIGHT, E.P., WILLEMS, C., ZEIJLMAKER, W.P., and JANSSEN, M.C. (1982) J. Immunol. *128*, 2539.

BALL, E.D., GRAZIANO, R.F., SHEN, L. and FANGER, M.W. (1982) Proc. Natl. Acad. Sci. (U.S.A.) *79*, 5374.

BARNES, D. and SATO, G. (1980) Cell *22*, 649.

BASCH, R.S., BERMAN, J.W. and LAKOW, E. (1983) J. Immunol. Meth. *56*, 269.

BATTEIGER, B., NEWHALL, W.J. and JONES, R.B. (1982) J. Immunol. Meth. *55*, 297.

BAYER, E.A. and WILCHEK, M. (1980) Meth. Biochem. Anal. *26*, 1.

BAZIN, H., BECKERS, A., DECKERS, C. and HEREMANS, J.F. (1972) Eur. J. Cancer *10*, 568.

BAZIN, H., BECKERS, A., DECKERS, C. and MORIAME, M. (1973) J. Natl. Cancer Inst. *51*, 1359.

BAZIN, H. (1982) in: Protides of the Biological Fluids, 29th Colloquium, Ed. Peeters, H., Pergamon, p. 615.

BAZIN, H. (1983) Personal communication.

BEEZLEY, B. and RUDDLE, N.H. (1982) J. Immunol. Meth. *52*, 269.

BEGENT, R.J.H., KEEP, P.A., GREENE, A.J., SEARLE, F., BAGEHAWE, K.D., JEWKES, R.F., JONES, B.E., BARRATT, G.M. and RYMAN, B.E. (1982) Lancet, October 2nd.

BENNET, F.C. and YEOMAN, C. (1983) J. Immunol. Meth. *61*, 201.

BERKOWITZ, D.B. and WEBERT, D.W. (1981) J. Immunol. Meth. *47*, 121.

BERZOFSKY, J. (1983) Immunol. Today *4*, 299.

BEVERLEY, P.C.L. (1982) Nature *297*, 358.

BHORJEE, J.S., BARCLAY, S.L., WEDRYCHOWSKI, A. and SMITH, A.M. (1983) J. Cell. Biol. *97*, 389.

BISCHOFF, R., EISERT, R.M., SCHEDEL, I., VIENKEN, J. and ZIMMERMEN, U. (1982) FEBS Lett. *147*, 64.

BLAIR, A.H. and GHOSE, T.I. (1983) J. Immunol. Meth. *59*, 129.

BLOOM, A.D. and NAKAMURA, F.T. (1974) Proc. Natl. Acad. Sci. (U.S.A.) *71*, 2689.

BLOW, A.M.J., BOTHAM, G.M., FISHER, D., GOODALL, A.H., TILCOCK, C.P.S. and LUCY, J.A. (1978) FEBS Lett. *94*, 305.

BRODIN, T., OLSSON, L. and SJOGREN, H. (1983) J. Immunol. Meth. *60*, 1.

BRODSKY, F.M., PARHAM, P., BARNSTABLE, C.J., CRUMPTON, M.J. and BODMER, W.F. (1979) Immunol. Rev. *47*, 3.

BRUCK, C., PORTELLE, D., GLINER, R.C. and BOLLEN, A. (1982) J. Immunol. Meth. *53*, 313.

BRUINS, S.C., INGWER, I., ZECKEL, M.I. and WHITE, A.C. (1978) Infect. Immunol. *21*, 721.

BURNET, F.M. (1959) The Clonal Section Theory of Acquired Immunity. Cambridge University Press.

BUTCHER, E.C. and WEISSMAN, I.L. (1980) J. Immunol. Meth. *37*, 97.

CARROLL, S.B. and STOLLAR, B.D. (1982) Proc. Natl. Acad. Sci. (U.S.A.) *79*, 7233.

CHALON, M.P., MILNE, R.W. and VAERMAN, J.P. (1979) Scand. J. Immunol. 9, 359.

CIVIN, C.I. and BANQUERIGO, M.L. (1983) J. Immunol. Meth. *61*, 1.

CLAFLIN, L. and WILLIAMS, K. (1978) Curr. Top. Micro. Immunol. *81*, 107.

CLARK, M., COBBOLD, S., HALE, G. and WALDMAN, H. (1983) Immunol. Today *4*, 100.

CLARK, W.A., FROGNER, K.S. and ZAK, R. (1982) J. Cell. Biol. *95*, 369a.

COFFINO, P., KNOWLES, B., NATHENSON, S.G. and SCHARFF, M.D. (1971) Nature, New Biol. *231*, 87.

COLWELL, D.E., GOLLAHON, K.A., McGHEE, J.R. andMICHALEK, S.M. (1982) J. Immunol. Meth. *54*, 259.

COTE, R.J. MORRISSEY, D.M., HOUGHTON, A.N., BEATTIE, E.J., OETTGEN, H.F. and OLD, L.J. (1983) Proc. Natl. Acad. Sci. (U.S.A.) *80*, 2026.

COTE, R.J., MORRISEY, D.M., HOUGHTON, A.M., BEATTIE, E.J., OETTGEN, H.F. and OLD, L.J. (983) Proc. Natl. Acad. Sci. (U.S.A.) *80, 2026.

COTTON, R.G.H. and MILSTEIN, C. (1973) Nature *244*, 42.

COX, R. and MASSON, W. (1978) Nature *276*, 629.

CRAWFORD, D., BARLOW, N.S., HARRISON, J.F., WINGER, L. and HUEKINS, E.R. (1982) Lancet *i*, No. 8321, 386.

CRAWFORD, D.H., HUEHNS, E.R. and EPSTEIN, M.A. (1983) Lancet, 7th May, 1040.

CROCE, C.M. and KOPROWSKI, H. (1974) J. Exp. Med. *139*, 1350.

CROCE, C.M., LINNENBACH, A., HALL, W., STEPLEWSKI, Z. and KOPROWSKI, H. (1980) Nature *288*, 488.

CROCE, C.M., SHANDER, M., MARTINIS, J., CICUREL, L., D'ANCONA, G.G. and

KOPROWSKI, H. (1980) Eur. J. Immunol. *10*, 486.

DANGL, J.L. and HERZENBERG, L.A. (1982) J. Immunol. Meth. *52*, 1.

DAVIDSON, R.L., O'MALLEY, K.A. and WHEELER, T.B. (1976) Som. Cell Gen. *2*. 271.

DAVIES, A.J.S. and CRUMPTON, M.J. (Eds.) (1982) Experimental approaches to drug targetting. Cancer Surveys Vol. 1.

DAVIS, J.M., PENNINGTON, J.E., KUBLER, A.M. and CONSCIENCE, J.F. (1982) J. Immunol. Meth. *50*, 161.

DE BLAS, A.L., RATNAPARKHI, M.V. and MOSIMANN, J.E. (1981) J. Immunol. Meth. *45*, 109.

DOUILLARD, J.Y., HOFFMAN, T. and HERBERMAN, R.B. (1980) J. Immunol. Meth. *39*, 309.

DUHAMEL, R.C., SCHUR, P.H., BRENDEL, K. and MEEZAN, E. (1979) J. Immunol. Meth. *31*, 211.

EDWARDS, P.A.W. (1981) Biochem. J. *200*, 1.

EDWARDS, P.A.W., SMITH, C.M., MUNRO NEVILLE, A. and O'HARE, M.J. (1982) Eur. J. Immunol. *12*, 641.

EDWARDS, P.A.W., and O'HARE, M.J. (1984) in: Methods in Haematology. Ed. Beverley, P. Churchill–Livingstone.

EHRLICH, P., MOYLE, W.R., MOUSTAFA, Z.A. and CANFIELD, R.E. (1982) J. Immunol. *128*, 2709.

EILAT, D. (1982) Mol. Immunol. *19*, 943.

EISENBARTH, G.S. (1981) Anal. Biochem. *111*, 1.

ENGVALL, E. and PERLMAN, P. (1971) Immunochemistry *8*, 871.

ENGVALL, E. and PESCE, A.J. (Eds.) (1978) Quantitative Immunoassay, Scand. J. Immunol., Suppl. 7.

ENGVALL, E. (1981) Meth. Enzymol. *70*.

EPENETOS, A.A., BRITTON, K.E., MATHER, S., SHEPHERD, J., GRANOWSKA, M., TAYLOR-PAPDIMITROU, J., NIMMON, C.C., DURBIN, H., HAWKINS, L.R., MALPAS, J.S. and BODMER, W.F. (1982) Lancet, 6th Nov.

ERIKSON, J., MARTINIS, J. and CROCE, C.M. (1981) Nature *294*, 173.

EVANS, H.J. and VIJAYALAXMI (1981) Nature *292*, 601.

EY, P.L., PROWSE, S.J. and JENKIN, C.R. (1978) Immunochem. *15*, 429.

FARR, A.G. and NAKANE, P.K. (1981) J. Immunol. Meth. *47,* 129.

FATHMAN, C.G. and FITCH, F.W. (Eds.) (1982) Isolation, Characterisation and Utilisation of T Lymphocyte Clones. Academic Press, New York.

FAZEKAS DE ST GROTH, S.J. and SCHEIDEGGER, D. (1980) J. Immunol. Meth. *35*,1.

FAZEKAS DE ST GROTH, S.J. (1983) J. Immunol. Meth. *57*, 121.

FELLOWS, R.E. and EISENBARTH, G.S. (1981) Monoclonal Antibodies in Endocrine Research, Raven Press, New York.

FERGUSON, M., SCHILD, G.C., MINAR, P.D., YATES, P.J. and SPITZ, M. (1982) J. Gen. Virol. *54*, 437.

FESTING, M.F.W. (1979) Inbred Strains in Biomedical Research. Macmillan Press.

FIELDS, E.A., DAVIS, C.L., DREESMAN, G.R., BRADLEY, D.W. and MAYNARD, J.E. (1981) J. Immunol. Meth. *47*, 145.

FINN, O.J., BONIVER, J. and KAPLAN, H.S. (1979) Proc. Natl. Acad. Sci. (U.S.A.) *76*, 4033.

FOGH, J. and HACKER, C. (1960) Exp. Cell. Res. *21*, 242.

FOGH. J. and FOGH, H. (1968) Proc. Soc. Exp. Biol. Med. *117*, 899.

FOUNG, S.K.H., SASKI, D.T., GRUMET, F.C. and ENGLEMAN, E.G. (1982) Proc. Natl. Acad. Sci. (U.S.A.) *79*, 484.

FOX, R.M., TRIPP, E.H. and TATTERSALL, M.H.N. (1980) Cancer Res. *40*, 1718.

FRANKEL, M.E. and GERHARD, W. (1979) Mol. Immunol. *16*, 101.

FRASER, R.H., MUNRO, A.C., WILLIAMSON, A.R., BARNE, E.K., HAMILTON, E.A. and MITCHELL, R. (1982) J. Immunoget. *9*, 303.

FRIGUET, B., DJAVADI-OHANIANCE, L., PAGES, J., BUSSARD, A. and GOLDBERG, M. (1983) J. Immunol. Meth. *60*, 351.

GALFRE, G. and MILSTEIN, C. (1981) Methods in Enzymology, p. 738 Eds. Langone and Van Vanukis, H., Gen. Eds. Colowick, S.P. and Kaplan, N.O.

GALFRE, G. and CLARK, M.R. (1981) In Monoclonal Antibodies and Developments in Immunoassay, Eds. Albertini, A. and Ekins, R., Elsevier.

GALFRE, G., MILSTEIN, C. and WRIGHT, B. (1979) Nature *277*, 131.

GALFRE, G., HOWE, S.C., MILSTEIN, C., BUTCHER, G.W. and HOWARD, J.C. (1977) Nature *266*, 550.

GERSON, J.A., BEVERLEY, P.C.L., COAKHAM, H.B. and HARPER, E.I. (1982) Nature *298*, 375.

GEFTER, M.L., MARGULIES, D.H. and SCHARFF, M.D. (1977) Somatic Cell Genet. *3*, 231.

GERHARD, W., YEWDALL, J., FRENKEL, M.E. and WEBSTER, R. (1981) Nature *290*, 713.

GIGLOTTI, F. and INSEI, R. (1982) J. Clin. Invest. *70*, 1306.

GILLILAND, D.G., STEPLEWSKI, Z., COLLIER, R.J., MITCHELL, K.F., CHENG, T.H. and KOPROWSKI, H. (1980) Proc. Natl. Acad. Sci. (U.S.A.) *77*, 4539.

GIALLONGO, G., KOUCHOUMIAN, L. and KING, T.P. (1982) J. Immunol. Meth. *52*, 379.

GLASSY, M.C., HANDLEY, H., STRAYER, D., LOWE, H., ASTARITA, R. and ROYSTON, I. (1983) Fed. Proc. *42*, 402.

GLASSY, M.C., HANDLEY, H.H., HAGIWARA, H. and ROYSTON, R. (1983) Proc. Natl. Acad. Sci. (U.S.A.) *80*, 6327.

GODING, J.W. (1976) J. Immunol. Meth. *52*, 379.

GODING, J.W. (1978) J. Immunol. Meth. *20*, 241.

GODING, J.W. (1980) J. Immunol. Meth. *39*, 285.

GOLDSBY, R.A., OSBORNE, B.A., SIMPSON, E. and HERZENBERG, L.A. (1977) Nature *267*, 707.

GRAY, B. (1979) J. Immunol. Meth. *28*, 187.

GREAVES, M.F. and BROWN, G. (1974) J. Immunol. *112*, 420.

GREY, H.M., HIRST, J.W. and COHN, M. (1971) J. Exp. Med. *133*, 289.

GUTMAN, G.A., WARNER, N.L., HARRIS, A.W. and BOWLES, A. (1978) J. Immunol. Meth. *21*, 101.

HAAKE, D.A., FRANKLIN, E.C. and FRANGIONE, B. (1982) J. Immunol. *129*, 190.

HAAS, W. and VON BOEHMER, H. (1982) J. Immunol. Meth. *52*, 137.

HABER, E., KATUS, H., HURRELL, J., MATSUEDA, G., EHRLICH, P., ZURAWSKI, F.R. and KHAW, B. (1982) J. Mol. Cell. Cardiol. *14*, Suppl. 3, 139.

HAMBLIN, T.J., ABDUL-AHAD, A.K., GORDON, J., STEPHENSON, F.K. and STEPHEN-
SON, G.T. (1980) Brit. J. Cancer *42*, 495.

HANES, B.D. and RICKWOOD, D. (Eds.) (1981) Gel Electrophoresis of Proteins. IRC
Press.

HAMMERLING, G.J., HAMMERLING, U. and KEARNEY, J.F. (1981) Monoclonal Antibodies and T cell hybridomas. Elsevier.

HARRIS, H. (1970) Cell Fusion. The Dunham Lectures. Oxford University Press.

HARRIS, H. and WATKINS, J.F. (1975) Nature *205*, 640.

HAWKES, B., NIDDAY, B. and GORDON, J. (1982) Anal. Biochem. *119*, 142.

HENDRY, R.M. and HERRMAN, J.E. (1980) J. Immunol. Meth. *35*, 285.

HERBERT, W.J. (1973) Laboratory Animal Techniques for Immunologists, in:
Handbook of Experimental Immunology. Ed. Weir, D.M. Vol. 3, 2nd edn. Blackwell.

HEUSSER, C.H., STOCKER, J.W. and GISLER, R.H. (1981) Methods in Enzymology
73, 406. Ed. Langone, J.J. and Van Vanukis, H.

HILWIG, I. and GROPP, A. (1972) Exp. Cell Res. *75*, 122.

HOCH, S., SCHUR, P.H. and SCHWABER, J. (1983) Clin. Immunol. Immunopathol.
27, 28.

HOFFMAN, G.J., LAZAROWITZ, S.G. and HAYWARD, S.D. (1980) Proc. Natl. Acad.
Sci. (U.S.A.) *77*, 2979.

HOOGENRAD, N., HELMAN, T. and HOOGENRAD, J. (1983) J. Immunol. Meth. *61*,
317.

HOWARD, J.C., BUTCHER, G.W., GALFRE, G., MILSTEIN, C. and MILSTEIN, C.P.
(1979) Immunol. Rev. *47*, 137.

HOUBA, V. and CHAN, S.H. (Eds.) (1972) Properties of Monoclonal Antibodies
Produced by Hybridoma Technology and their Application to the Study of Human
Disease, Publ. UNDP/World Bank/WHO, Geneva.

HUET, J., SENTENAC, A. and FROMAGEOT, P. (1982) J. Biol. Chem. *257*, 2613.

HUGLE, B., GULDNER, H., BAUTZ, F.A. and ALONSO, A. (1982) Exp. Cell Res. *142*,
119.

HURWITZ, E., LEVY, R., MARON, R., WICHEK, M., ARNON, R. and SELA, M. (1975)
Cancer Res. *35*, 1175.

ILFELD, D.N., CATHCART, M.K., KRAKAUER, R.S. and BLAESE, M. (1981) Cell.
Immunol. *57*, 400.

IRIGOYEN, O., RIZZOLO, P.V., THOMAS, Y., ROGOZINSKI, L. and CHESS, L. (1981)
J. Exp. Med. *154*, 1827.

ISCOVE, N.N. and MELCHERS, F. (1978) J. Exp. Med. *147*, 923.

JANOSSY, G. (1982) Monoclonal Antibodies in Bone Marrow Transplantation, Proc.
Roy. Soc. Edin. *81B*, 233.

JANOSSY, G., COSIMI, A.B. and GOLDSTEIN, G. (1982) In Monoclonal Antibodies and
Clinical Medicine. Eds. Mcmichael, A. and Fabre, J.W., Academic Press.

JOHNSTONE, A. and THORPE, R. (1982) Immunochemistry in Practice. Blackwell.

JUY, D., BARBIER, E., LE GUERN, C. and CAZENAVE, P. (1982) J. Immunol. *129*,
115.

KAMO, I., FURUKAWA, S., TADA, A., MANO, YIWASAKI, YFRUSE, T., ITO, N.,
HAYASHI, K. and SATOYOSHI, E. (1982) Science *215*, 995.

KANE, C.M., CHENG, P.F., BURCH, J.B.E. and WEINTRAUB, H. (1982) Proc. Natl. Acad. Sci. (U.S.A.) *79*, 6265.

KAPLAN, M.E. and CLARK, C. (1974) J. Immunol. Meth. *5*, 131.

KAPP, J.A., ARANEO, B.A and CLEVINGER, B.L. (1980) J. Exp. Med. *152*, 235.

KAPPLER, J.W., SKIDMORE, B., WHITE, J. and MARRACK, P. (1981) J. Exp. Med. *153*, 1198.

KAPPLER, J., KUBO, R., HASKINS, K., WHITE, J. and MARRACK, D. (1983) Cell *34*, 727.

KARPAS, A., FISCHER, P. and SWIRSKY, D. (1982) Science *216*, 997.

KEARNEY, J.F., RADBRUCH, A., LEISGANG, B. and RAJEWSKY, K. (1979) J. Immunol. *123*, 1548.

KEMSHEAD, J.T., GOLDMAN, A., FRITSCHY, J., MALPAS, J.S. and PRITCHARD, J. (1983) Lancet 1st Jan.

KENNET, R.H., MCKEARN, R.J. and BECHTOL, K.B. (Eds.) (1980) Monoclonal Antibodies, Plenum Press.

KING, T.P. and KOCHOUMIAN, L. (1979) J. Immunol. Meth. *78*, 201.

KIOKE, T., NAGASAWA, R., NAGATA, N. and SHIRAI, T. (1982) Immunol. Lett. *4*, 93.

KLAUS, G.G.B., PEPYS, M.B., KITAJIMA, K. and ASKONAS, B.A. (1979) Immunology *38*, 687.

KLEBE, R.J. and MANCUSO, M.G. (1981) Somatic Cell Gen. *7*, 473.

KNUTTON, S. and PASTERNAK, C.A. (1979) Trends in Biochemical Sciences, 220.

KOBAYASHI, Y., ASADA, M., HIGUCHI, M. and OSAWA, T. (1982) J. Immunol. *128*, 2714.

KOHLER, G. and MILSTEIN, C. (1975) Nature *256*, 495.

KOHLER, G. and MILSTEIN, C. (1976) Eur. J. Immunol. *6*, 511.

KOHLER, G., HOWE, S.C. and MILSTEIN, C. (1976) Eur. J. Immunol. *6*, 292.

KOHLER, G., HENGARTNER, H. and SHULMAN, M. (1978) Eur. J. Immunol. *8*, 82.

KOMISAR, J.L., FUHRMAN, J.A. and CEBRA, J.J. (1982) J. Immunol. *128*, 2376.

KONTIAINEN, S., SIMPSON, E., BOHRER, E., BEVERLEY, P.C.L., HERZENBERG, L.A., FITZPATRICK, W.C., VOGT, P., TORANO, A., MCKENZIE, I.F.C. and FELDMAN, M. (1978) Nature *274*, 480.

KOO, G.C. and GOLDBERG, C. (1978) J. Immunol. Meth. *23*, 197.

KOZBOR, D. and RODER, J.C. (1981) J. Immunol. *127*, 1275.

KOZBOR, D. and RODER, J.C. (1983) Immunol. Today *4*, 72–79.

KOZBOR, D., LAGARDE, A.E. and RODER, J.C. (1982) Proc. Natl. Acad. Sci. (U.S.A.) 79, 6651.

KROLICK, K.A., VILLEMEZ, C., ISAKSON, P., UHR, J.W. and VITETTA, E.S. (1980) Proc. Natl. Acad. Sci. (U.S.A.) 77, 5419.

KRONVALL, G., GREY, H.M. and WILLIAMS, R.C. (1970) J. Immunol. *105*, 1116.

LABROUSSE, H., GUESDON, J., RAGIMBEAU, J. and AVRAMEAS, S. (1982) J. Immunol. Meth. *48*, 133.

LACHMANN, P.J., OLROYD, R.G., MILSTEIN, C. and WRIGHT, B.W. (1980) Immunology *43*, 503.

Lancet (1983) Editorial March 5th. Drug targeting in cancer.

LANE, H.C., VOLKMAN, D.J., WHALEN, G. and FAUCI, A.S. (1981) J. Exp. Med. *154*,

1043.

LANE, D. and KOPROWSKI, H. (1982) Nature *296*, 200.

LANGONE, J.J. (1982a) J. Immunol. Meth. *51*, 3.

LANGONE, J.J. (1982b) J. Immunol. Meth. *55*, 277.

LANGONE, J.J. and VAN VANUKIS, H. (1981, 1983) Methods in Enzymology, Vols. 73 and 92. Academic Press.

LEDBETTER, J.A. and HERZENBERG, L.A. (1979) Immunol. Rev. *47*, 63.

LEHTONEN, O. and VILJANEN, M.K. (1980a) J. Immunol. Meth. *34*, 61.

LEHTONEN, O. and VILJANEN, M.K. (1980b) J. Immunol. Meth. *36*, 63.

LENNOX, E.S. and SIKORA, K. (1982) in: McMichael and Fabre, Ch. 5.

LERNER, R.A. (1982) Nature *299*, 592.

LERNHARDT, W., Andersson, J., COUTHINO, A. and MELCHERS, F. (1978) Exp. Cell Res. *111*, 309.

LESERMAN, L.D., MACHY, P. and BARBET, J. (1981) Nature *293*, 226.

LITTLEFIELD, J.W. (1964) Science *145*, 709.

LITTLEFIELD, J.W. (1963) Proc. Natl. Acad. Sci. (U.S.A.) *50*, 568.

LOCKER, O. and MOTTA, G. (1983) J. Immunol. Meth. *59*, 269.

LONAI, P., BITTON, S., SAVELKOUL, H.F.J., PURI, J. and HAMMERLING, G.J. (1981) J. Exp. Med. *154*, 1910.

LOVBORG, U. (1982) Monoclonal Antibodies Production and Maintenance. Heinemann.

LUBBE, F.H., ROSSI, I.G. and ZAALBERG, O.B. (1976) J. Immunol. Meth. *12*, 131.

LUBEN, R.A. and MOHLER, M.A. (1980) Mol. Immunol. *17*, 635.

MCCONNELL, I., MUNRO, A. and WALDMAN, H. (1981) The Immune System, 2nd edn., Blackwell, Oxford.

MCCORMACK, M., DUNN, J.H.J. and CAMPBELL, A.M. (1982) J. Immunol. Meth. *49*, 151.

MCGEE, J.O., ASHALL, F., BRAMWELL, M.E., WOODS, J.C. and HARRIS, H. (1982) Lancet, 3rd July, p. 7.

MCMAHON-PRATT, D. and DAVID, J. (1981) Nature *284*, 366.

MCHUGH, Y.E., WALTHALL, B.J. and STEIMER. K.S. (1983) Biotechniques June/July, p. 72.

MCMICHAEL, A.J. and FABRE, J.W. (1982) Monoclonal Antibodies in Clinical Medicine, Academic Press, New York.

MARCUS, M., LAVI, U., NATTENBERG, A., ROTTEM, S. and MARKOWITZ, O. (1980) Nature *285*, 659.

MARGULIES, D.H., KUEHL, W.M. and SCHARFF, M.D. (1976) Cell *8*, 405.

MASON, D.W. and WILLIAMS, A.F. (1980) Biochem. J. *187*, 1.

MECHLINSKI, W. and SCHAFFNER, C.P. (1970) Tetrahedron Lett. *44*, 3873.

MEDGYESI, G.A., FUST, G., GERGELY, J. and BAZIN, H. (1978) Immunochem. *15*, 125.

MELDERS, F., POTTER, M. and WARNER, N.L. (Eds.) (1980) Lymphocyte hybridomas. Curr. Top. Micro. Immunol. *81*.

MILLER, G. and LIPMAN, M. (1973) Proc. Natl. Acad. Sci. (U.S.A.) *70*, 190.

MILLER, K.F., BOLT, D.J. and GOLDSBY, R.M. (1983) J. Immunol. Meth. *59*, 277.

MILLER, R.A., MALONEY, D.G., MCKILLOP, J. and LEVY, R. (1981) Blood *58*, 78.

MILLER, R.A., MALONEY, D.G., WARNKE, R. and LEVY, R. (1982) N. Engl. J. Med. 306, 517.

MILLER, T.J. and STONE, H.O. (1978) J. Immunol. Meth. 24, 111.

MILSTEIN, C. and CUELLO, A.C. (1983) Nature 305, 537.

MILSTEIN, C., WRIGHT, B. and CUELLO, A.C. (1983) Mol. Immunol. 20, 113.

MITCHELL, G.F. (1981) in: Proc. Symp. Monoclonal Abs and Disease, Eds. Houba, V. and Chan, S.H. Publ. UNDP/World Bank/WHO.

MOLDAY, R.S. and MACKENZIE, D. (1983) Biochemistry 22, 653.

MOLONEY, J.B. (1960) J. Natl. Canc. Inst. 24, 933.

MORI, T., KANO, K., MERRICK, J.M. and MILGROM, F. (1978) Cell. Immunol. 40, 28.

MORI, T., KANO, K., MERRICK, J. and MILGROM, F. (1981) Cell. Immunol. 58.

MOSMANN, T.R., GALLATIN, M. and LONGNECKER, B.M. (1980) J. Immunol. 125, 1152.

MURAGUCHI, A., KISHIMOTO, T., KURITANI, T. and YAMAMURA, Y. (1980) J. Immunol. 125, 2638.

MURAKAMI, H., MASUI, H., SATO, G.H., SUEOKA, N., CHOW, T.P. and KANO-SUEOKA, T. (1982) Proc. Natl. Acad. Sci. (U.S.A.) 79, 1158.

NADLER, L.M., STASHENKO, P., HARDY, R., KAPLAN, W.D., BUTTON, L.N., LUFE, D.W., ANTIMAN, K.H. and SCHLOSSMAN, S.F. (1980) Cancer Res. 40, 3147.

NARDONE, R.M., TODD, J., GONZALEZ, P. and GAFFNEY, E.V. (1965) Science 149, 1100.

NELSON, J.A., CARPENTER, J.W., ROSE, L.M. and ADAMSON, D.J. (1975) Cancer Res. 35, 2872.

NEWSOME-DAVIS, J. (1981) Immunol. Today 2, No. 2 (ii–iv).

NICOLOTTI, R.A., BRILES, D.E., SCHROER, J.A. and DAVIE, J.M. (1980) J. Immunol. Meth. 33, 101.

NILSSON, R., MRHRE, E., KRONVALL, G. and SJOGREN, H.O. (1982) Mol. Immunol. 19, 119.

NORWOOD, T.H., ZIEGLER, C.J. and MARTIN, G.M. (1976) Somatic Cell Genet. 2, 263.

NOSSAL, J.G. and PIKE, B. (1976) Immunology 30, 189.

OI, V.T., JONES, P.P., GODING, J.W., HERZENBERG, L.A. and HERZENBERG, L.A. (1978) Curr. Top. Microbiol. Immunol. 81, 115.

OKADA, M., YOSHIMURA, N., KAIEDA, T., YAMAMURA, Y. and KISHIMOTO, T. (1981) Proc. Natl. Acad. Sci. (U.S.A.) 78, 7717.

OLIVER, D.G., SANDERS, A.H., HOGG, R.D. and HELLMAN, J.W. (1981) J. Immunol. Meth. 42, 195.

OLSSON, L. and KAPLAN, H.S. (1980) Proc. Natl. Acad. Sci. (U.S.A.) 77, 5429.

OLSSON, L., KRONSTROM, H., CAMBON-DE MOUZON, A., HONSIK, C., BRODIN, T. and JAKOBSEN, B. (1983) J. Immunol. Meth. 61, 17.

O'SULLIVAN, M.J. and MARKS, V. (1981) Meth. Enzymol. 73, 147.

PACIFICO, A. and CAPRA, J.D. (1980) J. Exp. Med. 152, 1289.

PARDUE, R.L., BRADY, R.C., PERRY, G.W. and DEDMAN, J.R. (1983) J. Cell. Biol. 96, 1149.

PARHAM, P., ANDROLEWICZ, M.J., BRODSKY, F.M., HOLMES, N.J. and WAYS, J.P.

(1982) J. Immunol. Meth. *53*, 133.

PARKS, D.R., BRYAN, V.M. OI, V.T. and HERZENBERG, L.A. (1979) Proc. Natl. Acad. Sci. (U.S.A.) *76*, 1962.

PEARSON, T.W. (1982) Properties of MCAs and Specificities, in: Houba, V. and Chan, S.H. (Eds.) (see above) Chapter 2.

PEETERS, H. (Ed.) (1982) Protides of the Biological Fluids, *30*.

PEREIRA, K., KLASSEN, T. and BARING, J.R. (1980) Inf. Immunol. *29*, 724.

PESCE, A.J., FORD, D.J., GAIZUTIS, M. and POLLACK, V.E. (1978) in: Quantitative Immunoassay, Eds. Engvall, E. and Pesce, A.J., Scand. J. Immunol. Suppl. 7.

PHILLIPS, J., SIKORA, K. and WATSON, J.V. (1982) Lancet, Nov. 27th, p. 1215.

PICKERING, J.W. and GELDER, F.B. (1982) J. Immunol. *128*, 406.

PIERSBACHER, M.D., HAYMAN, E.G. and RUOSLAHTI, E. (1981) Cell *26*, 259.

PINTUS, C., RANSOME, J.H. and EVANS, C.H. (1983) J. Immunol. Meth. *61*, 195.

POLLARD, K.M. and WEBB, J. (1982) J. Immunol. Meth. *54*, 81.

POLLOCK, M.E. and KENNY, G.E. (1963) Proc. Soc. Exp. Biol. Med. *112*, 176.

PONTECORVO, G. (1976) Somat. Cell. Genet. *1*, 397.

RAISON, R.L., WALKER, K.Z., HALNAN, C.R.E., BRISCOE, D. and BASTEN, A. (1982) J. Exp. Med. *156*, 1380.

READING, C.L. (1982) J. Immunol. Meth. *53*, R1.

REMMERS, E.F., COLWELL, R.R. and GOLDSBY, R.A. (1982) Inf. Immunol. *37*, 70.

RENER, J., CARTER, R., ROSENBERG, Y. and MILLER, L.H. (1980) Proc. Natl. Acad. Sci. (U.S.A.) *77*, 6797.

RICCIARDI-CASTAGNOLI, A., DORIA, G. and ADORINI, L. (1981) Proc. Natl. Acad. Sci. (U.S.A.) *78*, 3804.

RICHARDS, F.F., KONIGSBERG, W.H., ROSENSTORN, R.W. and VORGA, J.M. (1975) Science *187*, 130.

RICHMAN, D., CLEVELAND, P., OXMAN, M., VAN WYKE, K. and WEBSTER, R. (1981) Proc. 5th Int. Congress Virol. Strasbourg.

RIGHETTI, P.G. (1983) Isoelectric Focusing, Theory, Methodology and Applications, in: Laboratory Techniques in Biochemistry, Eds. Work, T.S. and Burdon, R.H., Elsevier, Amsterdam.

RINGERTZ, N. and SAVAGE, R.E. (1976) Cell Hybrids, Academic Press, New York.

RITZ, J., BAST, R.C., CLAVELL, L.A., HERCEND, T., SALLAN, S.E., LIPTON, J.M., FEENEY, M. and SCHLOSSMAN, S.F. (1982) Lancet, July 10th, p. 60.

RITZ, J., PESONDO, J.M., SALLAN, S.G., CLAVELL, C.A., NOTIS-MCCONARTY, J., ROSENTHAL, P. and SCHLOSSMAN, S.F. (1981) Blood *58*, 141.

RÖDWELL, J.D., GEARHARDT, P.J. and KARUSH, F. (1983) J. Immunol. *130*, 313.

ROITT, I. (1980) Essential Immunology, 4th edn., Blackwell, Oxford.

ROSEN A., EK, K. and AMAN, P. (1979) J. Immunol. Meth. *28*.

ROSENBERG, Y. (1981) Cell. Immunol. *61*, 416.

ROUSSEAUX, J., PICQUE, M.T., BAZIN, H. and BISERTE, G. (1981) Mol. Immunol. *18*, 639.

ROWE, D.A. (1980) Immunology Today *1*, 30.

RUDDLE, F.H. and KUCHERLAPALI, R.S. (1974) Sci. Am. *231*, 36.

RUDDLE, F.H. and CONTA, B.S. (1982) Curr. Top. Microscop. Immunol. *100*, 239.

RUSSELL, W.C., NEWMAN, C. and WILLIAMSON, D.H. (1975) Nature *253*, 461.

SAABE, L.J.M., DeBODE, L. and VAN ROOD, J.J. (1983) J. Immunol. Meth. *57*, 21.

SAWMWEBER, H., SYMMONS, P., KABISCH, R., WILL, H. and BONHOEFFER, F. (1980) Chromosoma *80*, 253.

SCHLOM, J., WUNDERLICH, D. and TERAMOTO, Y.A. (1980) Proc. Natl. Acad. Sci. (U.S.A.) *77*, 6841.

SCHOENFELD, Y., YSU-LIN, S.G., GABRIELS, J.E., SILBERSTEIN, L.E., FURIE, B., STOLLAR, B.D. and SCHWARZ, R.S. (1982) J. Clin. Invest. *70*, 205.

SCHOENFELD, Y., ISENBERG, D.A., RAUCH, J., MADAIO, M.P., STOLLAR. B.D. and SCHWARTZ, R.S. (1983) J. Exp. Med. *158*, 718.

SCHOENFELD, D.Y., RAUCH, J., MASSICOTE, H., SYAMAL, K.D., AMNDRE-SCHWARZ, J. and STOLLAR, B.D. (1983) N. Eng. J. Med. *308*, 414.

SCHWABER, J. and COHEN, E.P. (1974) Proc. Natl. Acad. Sci. (U.S.A.) *71*, 2203.

SCHIMMELPFENG, L., LANGENBERG, U. and PETERS, J.H. (1980) Nature *285*, 661.

SCRIBNER, D.J. and MOORHEAD, J.W. (1982) J. Immunol. *128*, 1377.

SECHER, D.S. and BURKE, D.C. (1980) Nature *285*, 446.

SECHER, D.S., MILSTEIN, C. and ADETUGBO, K. (1977) Immunol. Rev. *36*, 51.

SHALEV, A., GREENBERG, A.H. and MCALPINE, P.J. (1980) J. Immunol. Meth. *38*, 125.

SHARON, J., KABAT, E.A. and MORRISON, S.L. (1982) Mol. Immunol. *19*, 389.

SHIH, W.J., COLE, P.J., DAPOLITO, G.M. and GERIN, J.L. (1980) J. Virol. Meth. *1*, 257.

SHULMAN, M., WILDE, C.D. and KOHLER, G. (1978) Nature *276*, 269.

SINCOVIRS, J.G., SHIRATO, E., GYROKY, F. CABINESS, J.R. and HOWE, C.D. (1970) in: Leukemia Lymphoma, Yearbook Med. Publ., Chicago.

SINGH, V.K. (1982) J. Immunol. Lett. *4*, 317.

SIPPEL, J.E., WEISS, H.K., JOSEF, S.W. and BESSLEY, W.J. (1978) J. Clin. Microbiol. *7*, 372.

SMITH, E., ROBERTS, K., BUTCHER, G. and GALFRE, G. (1984) Anal. Biochem., in press.

SMITH, M.A., CLEGG, J.A., SNARY, D. and TREJDOSIEWICZ, A.J. (1982) Parasitology *84*, 93.

SMITH, P.F. (1971) The Biology of Mycoplasmas, Academic Press, New York.

SOUTHERN, E. (1965) J. Mol. Biol. *98*, 503.

SPRINGER, T., GALFRE, G., SECHER, D.S. and MILSTEIN, C. (1978) E.J. Immunol. *8*, 539.

SREDNI, B., SIEKMANN, D.G., KUMAGAI, S., HOUSE, S., GREEN, I. and PAUL, W.E. (1981) J. Exp. Med. *154*, 1500.

STAHLI, C., STAEHELIN, T., MIGGIANO, V., SCHMIDT, J. and HARING, P. (1980) J. Immunol. Meth. *32*, 297.

STAINES, N.A. and LEW, A.M. (1980) Immunology, 40, 287.

STANISLAWSKI, M. and MITARD, M. (1976) Immunochemistry *13*, 979.

STEINITZ, M., IZAK, G., SNARY, D. and FLECHNER, I. (1980), Nature *287*, 443.

STEINITZ, M. and TAMIR, S. (1982) Eur. J. Immunol. *2*, 126.

STETLER, D.A., ROSE, K.M., WENGER, M.E., BERLIN, C.M. and JACOB, S.T. (1982) Proc. Natl. Acad. Sci. (U.S.A.) *79*, 7499.

STEWARD, M.W. (1978) in: Weir, D.M., Handbook of Experimental Immunology, 3rd edn., Blackwell, Oxford, Chapter 16.

STEWARD, Mj.J. (1977) in: Immunology, An advanced Textbook, Eds. Glynn, M.E. and Steward, M.W., Chapter 7, Wiley, New York.

SUTER, L., BRUGGEN, J. and SORG, C. (1980) J. Immunol. Meth. *39*, 407.

TAN, E.M. (1982) Adv. Immunol. *33*, 167.

TANIGUCHI, M. and MILLER, J.F.A.P. (1978) J. Exp. Med. *148,* 373.

TAUSSIG, M.J., HOLLIMAN, A. and WRIGHT, L.J. (1980) Immunology *39*, 57.

TAYLOR, D.W. and BUTTERWORTH, A.E. (1982) Parasitology *84*, 83.

TAYLOR-PAPADIMITRIOU, J., PETERSON, J.A., ARKLIE, J., BURCHELL, J., CARIANI, R.C., and BODMER, W.F. (1981) Int. J. Cancer *28*, 17.

THOMSON, R.J. (1982) Trends Biochem. Sci., *7*, 419.

TONEGAWA S. (1983) Nature *302*, 575.

TOWBIN, H., STAEHELIN, T. and GORDON, J. (1979) Proc. Natl. Acad. Sci. (U.S.A.) *76*, 4350.

TRACY, R.P., PATZMAN, J.A., KUMBURGER, P.K., HURST, J.A. and YOUNG, D.S. J. Immunol. Meth. *65*, 97.

TRUCCO, M.M., GAROTTA, G., STOCKER, J.W. and CEPPELLINI, R. (1979) Immunol. Rev. *47*, 219.

TROWBRIDGE, I. (1978) J. Exp. Med. *148*, 313.

TSU, T.T. and HERZENBERG, L.A. (1980) in: Selected Methods in Cell Immunology, Eds. Mishell, B.B. and Shigi, S.M., Freeman, San Francisco. p. 373.

TUNG, A.S. (1983) in: Methods in Enzymology, Vol. 92, Eds. Langone, J. and Van Vanukis, H. Academic Press, p. 47.

TURNER, B.M. (1981) Eur. J. Cell Biol. *24*, 266.

UNDERWOOD, P.A., KELLY, J.F., HARMAN, D.F. and MacMILLAN, H.M. (1983) J. Immunol. Meth. *60*, 33.

VOLLER, A., BARTLETT, A. and BIDWELL, D. (1981) Immunoassays for the 80s.

VONKE, V. and HIRSCH, I. (1982) Prog. Med. Virol. *28*, 146.

WALDOR, M.K., SRIRAM, S., McDEVITT, H.O. and STEINMAN, L. (1983) Proc. Natl. Acad. Sci. (U.S.A.) *80*, 2713.

WALKER, S.M., MEINKE, G.C. and WEIGLE, W.O. (1977) J. Exp. Med. *146*, 445.

WANDS, J.R., CARLSON, R.I., SCHOEMAKER, J., ISSELBACHER, K.J. and ZURAWSKI, V.R. (1981) Proc. Natl. Acad. Sci. (U.S.A.) *78*, 1214.

WARENIUS, H.M., TAYLOR, J.W., DURACK, B.E. and CROSS, P.A. (1983) Eur. J. Clin. Oncol. *19*, 547.

WATANABE, T., YOSHIZAKI, K., YAGURA, T. and YAMAMURA, Y. (1974) J. Immunol. *113*, 608.

WEETMAN, A.P., McGREGOR, A.M. and HALL, R. (1982) J. Immunol. Meth. *54*, 47.

WEIR, D.M. (Ed.) (1978) Handbook of Experimental Immunology, 3rd edn., Blackwell, Oxford.

WEISSMAN, I.L., HOOD, L.E. and WOOD, W.B. (1978) Essential Concepts in Immunology. Benjamin/Cummings.

WELLS, D.E. and PRICE, P.J. (1983) J. Immunol. Meth. *59*, 49.

WHITE, J. and HELENIUS, A. (1980) Proc. Natl. Acad. Sci. (U.S.A.) *77*, 3273.

WIKTOR, T.J. and KOPROWSKI, H. (1979) Proc. Natl. Acad. Sci. (U.S.A.) *75*, 3938.

WILLIAMS, C.A. and CHASE, M.W. (1967) Methods in Immunology and Immunochemistry, Vol. 1, Academic Press, New York.

WINGER, L., WINGER, C., SHASTRY, P., RUSSELL, A. and LONGNECKER, M. (1983) Proc. Natl. Acad. Sci. (U.S.A.) *80*, 4484.

WRIGHT, W.E. (1978) Exp. Cell Res. *112*, 395.

YELTON, D.E. and SCHARFF, M.D. (1981) Annu. Rev. Biochem. *50*, 657.

YOSHIDA, N., NUSSENZWEIG, R.S., POTOCNJAK, P., NUSSENWEIG, V. and AIKAWA, M. (1980) Science *207*, 71.

YOULE, R.J. and NEVILLE, D.M. (1980) Proc. Natl. Acad. Sci. (U.S.A.) *77*, 5483.

YURCHENKO, P.D., SPEICHER, D.W., MORROW, J.S., KNOWLES, W.J. and MAR-CHESI, V.T. (1982) J. Biol. Chem. *257*, 9103.

ZAGURY, D., PHALENTE, L., BERNARD, J., HOLLANDE, E. and BUTTING, G. (1979) Eur. J. Immunol. *9*, 1.

ZIEGLER, A. and HENGARTNER, H. (1977) Eur. J. Immunol. *7*, 690.

ZIOLA, B.R., MATIKAINEN, M.T. and SALMI, A. (1977) J. Immunol. Meth. *17*, 309.

ZWEIG, M., HEILMAN, C.J., RABIN, H., HOPKINS, R.F., NAUBAUER, R.H. and HEMPER, B. (1979) J. Virol. *32*, 676.

Addendum

General

A further volume of *Advances in Enzymology* (Langone and Van Vanukis, 1983) is now in circulation. Essentially it describes refinements in cloning and assay techniques. In particular the various assay techniques which have worked for various authors with specific antigens are given much coverage. There is also a large section on computer analysis of data at the end.

Sections which may have general application are referred to in the Addendum and in the main text.

Chapter 1

In tumour therapy, interesting data have been reported by Koprowski et al. (1983) who have found rodent monoclonal antibodies more effective than anticipated in human tumour therapy. They attribute their data to the production of anti-iodiotype antibodies in the patients which act as internal images of the tumour antigens and thus stimulate the human immune response.

The T lymphocyte receptor DNA clones (Section 1.3.5) are now being further characterized as predicted (Hedrick et al., 1984).

Chapter 2

The main changes here involve the rapid growth of the dot blotting technique (Section 2.6.10). A special apparatus for this is now marketed by BioRad and BRL (merging with Gibco U.K. to form a company called Life Technologies). Testing of these kits against ELISA in our laboratory has shown limited extra sensitivity despite the high capacity of nitrocellulose for most antigens. In addition, each kit which costs £ 300 is only equivalent to a single ELISA plate which means that a very large number a required for a wide screen. The kits give a very high background unless washed with non-ionic detergent (i.e. Tween 20 or Triton X-100) which may inhibit some detecting enzymes. Sera are often detected by them but monoclonal antibodies are detected less readily. The firms are usually very helpful about lending the kits for testing before purchase if the intentions are genuine. Before purchasing one, it is advisable to test it on an established *hybridoma* and not on serum. (See also Addendum to Chapter 10.)

Chapter 3

Rat hybridomas

The move to rat monoclonal antibodies is considerable, at least in the U.K. One problem has been the lack of convenient typing sera (Section 10.2) to the various rat IgG subclasses. Miles now market such antisera to the three rat IgG subclasses, inconveniently not all raised in the same species. It should be emphasised that polyclonal and *not* monoclonal typing antisera are preferable for this function.

Human cell lines

The WI-L2-729-HF$_2$ cell line is emerging as a good possible cell line for human fusions (Heitzman and Cohn, 1983; Edwards and O'Hare, 1984). It is reported to secrete low amounts of the parent immunoglobulin and high amounts of the specific immunoglobulin and to have remarkably high fusion frequencies. It is obtained from Dr. R. Lundak, Techniclone, 3301 South Harbor Boulevard, Santa Anna, CA 92704 (U.S.A.). However, it must be emphasised that no fully defined stable human monoclonal antibody has yet been produced from this or indeed most other human cell lines.

Chapter 4

There have been considerable advances in immunisation for specific isotypes and recalcitrant antigens. Adoptive transfer (Siriganian et al., 1983) is recommended in particular. In this technique a second, syngeneic, irradiated rodent is given both antigen and spleen cells from the first. It is a time-consuming and cumbersome technique which has proved of immense value in conventional immunology. It remains to be seen whether it will remain useful in view of the challenge of faster techniques such as in vitro immunisation (Section 4.3).

There has also been an increase in the number of papers which have utilised bands from both one- and two-dimensional PAGE for immunisation (Section 4.2). This is an extremely attractive possibility since it means that the immunising antigen is pure so that antiserum (or monoclonal antibodies) from such immunisations may yield pure antigen by affinity chromatography. Obviously such techniques may be refined to the point where antigen purification by column chromatography becomes obsolete.

Chapter 5

While more papers describing better feeder cells for human hybridomas in particular have appeared, no laboratory has produced hybridomas which justify their claims of superiority at this stage. Commercial claims should be examined sceptically and where possible, samples should be obtained for testing. A firm which is confident in its product will do this.

Chapter 7

There has been a definite shift of emphasis from transformation as such as a means of human hybridoma production to transformation as a means of stimulating cells to divide followed by fusion with a HAT-sensitive ouabain-resistant human myeloma line. This is claimed to stabilise the IgM antibodies often lost after some months of cloning in the transformation (EB system). There is no clear point in the transformation process where fusion yields optimal results but it is sensible to assume that this will be optimal after some preliminary cloning of transformed cells.

Chapter 10

The most relevant information in this section relates to epitope characterisation by (Western) immunoblotting (Section 10.4). Originally it was anticipated that this would be a very powerful tool in epitope analysis and spectacular success with clearly defined protein antigens has been achieved (e.g. Yurchenko et al., 1982). However, many laboratories have found difficulty in immunoblotting with *hybridomas* where serum blots give strong bands. The hybridomas perform well on ELISA but the immunoblot sensitivity is much lower. Additionally, the routine molecular weight standards run on a PAGE, often blot strongly on an enzyme immunoblot if they are tested for this as an antigen control.

The best approach to this problem at the moment is to run as pure an antigen as possible on PAGE to increase epitope density, test it against as high a concentration of monoclonal antibody as possible [i.e. ascites fluid (Section 9.3) or concentrated tissue culture supernatant (Section 9.6)], use amplification by multiple antibody sandwiches (i.e. antigen–mouse hybridoma–rabbit antimouse– goat anti rabbit with label) and vary the blocking conditions. Tween 20 as recommended by Batteiger et al. (1982) is an excellent blocking system for conventional serum but may mask the epitopes of some hybridomas so that adult serum or BSA blocking is a more suitable system. The initial tests recommended in Section 10.4 (dot blotting before electrophoresis) are particularly valuable in this respect.

Multiple band blotting of hybridomas also appears more and more frequently in the literature. As discussed in Section 10.4 this may reflect genuine polymorphism or proteolysis. It also definitely occurs with epitopes involving sugars and lipids. These move abnormally on protein electrophoreses.

In general, a carbohydrate epitope blots readily and a protein one less so.

References

BATTEIGER, B., NEWALL, W.J. and JONES, R.B. (1982) J. Immunol. Meth., *53,* 297.

EDWARDS, P.A.W. and O'HARE, M.J. (1984) in: Methods in Haematology. Ed. Beverley, P. Churchill–Livingstone.

HEDRICK, S.M., NEILSON, E.A., KAVALER, J., COHEN, D.I. and DAVIS, M.M. (1984) Nature *308,* 153.

HEITZMANN, J.G. and COHN, M. (1983) Mol. Biol. Med. *1,* 235.

KOPROWSKY, H., HERLYN, D., DEFREITAS, E., and SEARS, H.F. (1983) Proc. Natl. Acad. Sci. (U.S.A.) *81,* 216.

LANGONE, J. and VAN VANUKIS, H. (1983) (Eds.) Methods on Enzymology *93,* Academic Press.

SIRIGANIAN, R.P., FOX, P.C and BERENSTEIN, H. (1983) in: Methods in Enzymology Vol. 93, Eds. Langone, J. and Van Vanukis, H., p. 17.

YURCHENKO, P.D., SPEICHER, D.W., MORROW, J.S., KNOWLES, W.J. and MARCHESI, V.T. (1982) J. Biol Chem. *257,* 9103.

Subject index